T0362022

# Hyperhidrosis

*Editor*

PETER B. LICHT

# THORACIC SURGERY CLINICS

www.thoracic.theclinics.com

*Consulting Editor*
M. BLAIR MARSHALL

November 2016 • Volume 26 • Number 4

**ELSEVIER**

1600 John F. Kennedy Boulevard ● Suite 1800 ● Philadelphia, Pennsylvania, 19103-2899

http://www.thoracic.theclinics.com

**THORACIC SURGERY CLINICS Volume 26, Number 4**
**November 2016 ISSN 1547-4127, ISBN-13: 978-0-323-47695-9**

**Editor:** John Vassallo (j.vassallo@elsevier.com)
**Developmental Editor:** Susan Showalter

© **2016 Elsevier Inc. All rights reserved.**

This periodical and the individual contributions contained in it are protected under copyright by Elsevier, and the following terms and conditions apply to their use:

**Photocopying**

Single photocopies of single articles may be made for personal use as allowed by national copyright laws. Permission of the Publisher and payment of a fee is required for all other photocopying, including multiple or systematic copying, copying for advertising or promotional purposes, resale, and all forms of document delivery. Special rates are available for educational institutions that wish to make photocopies for non-profit educational classroom use. For information on how to seek permission visit www.elsevier.com/permissions or call: (+44) 1865 843830 (UK)/(+1) 215 239 3804 (USA).

**Derivative Works**

Subscribers may reproduce tables of contents or prepare lists of articles including abstracts for internal circulation within their institutions. Permission of the Publisher is required for resale or distribution outside the institution. Permission of the Publisher is required for all other derivative works, including compilations and translations (please consult www.elsevier.com/permissions).

**Electronic Storage or Usage**

Permission of the Publisher is required to store or use electronically any material contained in this periodical, including any article or part of an article (please consult www.elsevier.com/permissions). Except as outlined above, no part of this publication may be reproduced, stored in a retrieval system or transmitted in any form or by any means, electronic, mechanical, photo-copying, recording or otherwise, without prior written permission of the Publisher.

**Notice**

No responsibility is assumed by the Publisher for any injury and/or damage to persons or property as a matter of products liability, negligence or otherwise, or from any use or operation of any methods, products, instructions or ideas contained in the material herein. Because of rapid advances in the medical sciences, in particular, independent verification of diagnoses and drug dosages should be made.

Although all advertising material is expected to conform to ethical (medical) standards, inclusion in this publication does not constitute a guarantee or endorsement of the quality or value of such product or of the claims made of it by its manufacturer.

*Thoracic Surgery Clinics* (ISSN 1547-4127) is published quarterly by Elsevier Inc., 360 Park Avenue South, New York, NY 10010-1710. Months of publication are February, May, August, and November. Business and editorial offices: 1600 John F. Kennedy Boulevard, Suite 1800, Philadelphia, PA 19103-2899. Periodicals postage paid at New York, NY, and additional mailing offices. Subscription prices are $355.00 per year (US individuals), $501.00 per year (US institutions), $100.00 per year (US Students), $435.00 per year (Canadian individuals), $648.00 per year (Canadian institutions), $225.00 per year (Canadian and international students), $465.00 per year (international individuals), and $648.00 per year (international institutions). Foreign air speed delivery is included in all Clinics' subscription prices. All prices are subject to change without notice. **POSTMASTER:** Send address changes to Thoracic Surgery Clinics, Elsevier Health Sciences Division, Subscription Customer Service, 3251 Riverport Lane, Maryland Heights, MO 63043. **Customer Service (orders, claims, online, change of address): Telephone: 1-800-654-2452 (U.S. and Canada); 314-447-8871 (outside U.S. and Canada). Fax: 314-447-8029. E-mail: journalscustomerservice-usa@elsevier.com (for print support); journalsonlinesupport-usa@elsevier.com (for online support).**

*Reprints.* For copies of 100 or more, of articles in this publication, please contact Commercial Rights Department, Elsevier Inc., 360 Park Avenue South, New York, NY 10010-1710. Tel: 212-633-3874; Fax: 212-633-3820; E-mail: reprints@elsevier.com.

*Thoracic Surgery Clinics* is covered in *MEDLINE/PubMed (Index Medicus), EMBASE/Excerpta Medica, Science Citation Index Expanded (SciSearch®), Journal Citation Reports/Science Edition,* and *Current Contents®/Clinical Medicine*.

# Contributors

## CONSULTING EDITOR

**M. BLAIR MARSHALL, MD, FACS**
Chief, Division of Thoracic Surgery; Associate
Professor of Surgery, Department of Surgery,
Georgetown University Medical Center,
Georgetown University School of Medicine,
Washington, DC

## EDITOR

**PETER B. LICHT, MD, PhD**
Professor of Surgery, Department of
Cardiothoracic Surgery, Odense University
Hospital, Odense, Denmark

## AUTHORS

**ALAN EDMOND PARSONS CAMERON,
MA, MCh, FRCS**
Consultant Surgeon, Department of Surgery,
Ipswich Hospital, Ipswich, United Kingdom

**DROTT CHRISTER, MD, PhD**
Consultant Vascular Surgeon, Borås Hospital,
Borås, Sweden; Associate Professor of
Surgery, Sahlgrenska University, Gothenburg,
Sweden

**CLIFF P. CONNERY, MD**
Medical Director, Dyson Center for Cancer
Care, Thoracic Oncology, Vassar Brothers
Medical Center, Poughkeepsie, New York

**HUGO VEIGA SAMPAIO DA FONSECA, MD**
Thoracic Surgery Division, Heart Institute/
Clinics Hospital from University of São Paulo
Medical School, São Paulo, São Paulo, Brazil

**JOSÉ RIBAS MILANEZ DE CAMPOS,
MD, PhD**
Thoracic Surgeon, Division of Thoracic
Surgery, Hospital Israelita Albert Einstein;
Thoracic Surgeon, Division of Thoracic
Surgery, Heart Institute/Clinics Hospital,
University of São Paulo Medical School, São
Paulo, Brazil

**MALCOLM M. DeCAMP, MD**
Fowler McCormick Professor of Surgery;
Chief, Division of Thoracic Surgery,
Northwestern Memorial Hospital,
Northwestern University Feinberg School of
Medicine, Chicago, Illinois

**JULIANA MARIA FUKUDA, MD**
Fellow, Division of Vascular and Endovascular
Surgery, Hospital Israelita Albert Einstein,
São Paulo, Brazil

**DEE ANNA GLASER, MD**
Interim Chairman and Professor, Department
of Dermatology, Saint Louis University School
of Medicine, St Louis, Missouri

**LYALL A. GORENSTEIN, MD**
Assistant Clinical Professor of Surgery,
New York Presbyterian Hospital, Columbia
University, New York, New York

**MOSHE HASHMONAI, MD, FACS**
Retired Professor and Head, Department
of Surgery, Rambam Medical Center & Faculty
of Medicine, Technion – Israel Institute of
Technology, Haifa, Israel

**CONOR F. HYNES, MD**
Surgery Resident, Division of Thoracic
Surgery, Georgetown University Hospital,
Washington, DC

**MARK J. KRASNA, MD**
Corporate Medical Director of Oncology,
Meridian Cancer Care; Clinical Professor of
Surgery, Rutgers-Robert Wood Johnson
Medical School, Jersey Shore University
Medical Center, Neptune, New Jersey

**SMIDFELT KRISTIAN, MD**
Department of Vascular Surgery,
Sahlgrenska University Hospital, Gothenburg,
Sweden

**ANASTASIA O. KURTA, DO**
Clinical Research Fellow, Department of
Dermatology, Saint Louis University School of
Medicine, St Louis, Missouri

**M. BLAIR MARSHALL, MD, FACS**
Chief, Division of Thoracic Surgery; Associate
Professor of Surgery, Department of Surgery,
Georgetown University Medical Center,
Georgetown University School of Medicine,
Washington, DC

**ROMAN RIEGER, MD**
Department of Surgery,
Salzkammergut-Klinikum Gmunden,
Gmunden, Austria

**CHRISTOPH H. SCHICK, PD Dr**
Department of Surgery, University of
Erlangen-Nuremberg, Erlangen,
Germany

**JOEL M. STERNBACH, MD, MBA**
Bechily-Hodes Fellow in Esophagology,
Department of Surgery, Northwestern
University Feinberg School of Medicine,
Chicago, Illinois

**NELSON WOLOSKER, MD, PhD**
Vice President, Division of Vascular and
Endovascular Surgery, Albert Einstein
Israelite Hospital; Associate Professor,
Division of Vascular and Endovascular
Surgery, Clinics Hospital, University
of São Paulo Medical School, São Paulo,
Brazil

# Contents

Large case series and randomized trials over the past 25 years have consistently demonstrated thoracoscopic interruption of the sympathetic chain to be a safe and effective treatment of focal primary hyperhidrosis. The surgical technique has evolved toward less-invasive and less-extensive procedures in an effort to minimize perioperative morbidity and effectively balance postoperative compensatory sweating with symptomatic relief. This review summarizes available evidence regarding the surgical approach and the optimal level of interruption of the sympathetic chain based on a patient's presenting distribution of pathologic sweating.

Endoscopic thoracic sympathectomy (ETS) is an effective treatment of primary hyperhidrosis of the face, upper extremities, and axillae. The major limitation is the side effect of compensatory sweating severe enough that patients request reversal in up to 10% of cases. When ETS is performed by cutting the sympathetic chain, reversal requires nerve grafting. However, for ETS done with clips, reversal is a simple thoracoscopic outpatient procedure of removing the clips. Subsequent reversal of the sympathectomy, ie, nerve regeneration, is successful in many cases. However, follow-up is short. Factors contributing to success rates require further study.

 Video content accompanies this article at http://www.thoracic.theclinics.com.

There is a small subset of patients who have undergone endoscopic thoracic sympathectomy for hyperhidrosis or facial blushing who are dissatisfied and would wish reversal. Compensatory sweating is the most common side effect that causes a person to regret surgery. Treatment options are limited and usually not effective in patients with severe side effects from sympathectomy. Nerve graft interposition has been proven to be effective in experimental models and small clinical series. Da Vinci robotic nerve graft reconstruction with interposition graft and direct suturing of nerve and high magnification dissection most closely mirrors standard nerve reconstruction principles when done as a minimally invasive procedure.

The best way to evaluate the impact of primary hyperhidrosis on quality of life (QL) is through specific questionnaires, avoiding generic models that do not appropriately evaluate individuals. QL improves significantly in the short term after sympathectomy. In the longer term, a sustained and stable improvement is seen, although there is a small decline in the numbers; after 5 and even at 10 years of follow-up it shows virtually the same numerical distribution. Compensatory hyperhidrosis is a major side effect and the main aggravating factor in postoperative QL, requiring attention to its management and prevention.

Compensatory hyperhidrosis (HH) is the most common and feared side effect of thoracic sympathectomy, because patients with severe forms have their quality of life greatly impaired. The most well-known factors associated with compensatory HH are extension of manipulation of the sympathetic chain, level of sympathetic denervation, and body mass index. Technical developments as well as the proper selection of patients for surgery have been crucial in reducing the occurrence of severe forms of compensatory HH. Therapeutic options include topical agents, botulinum toxin, systemic anticholinergics, clip removal, and sympathetic chain reconstruction, although the efficacy is not well-established for all the methods.

Because of video-assisted thoracic technology and increased patient awareness of treatment options for palmar hyperhidrosis, endoscopic thoracic sympathectomy (ETS) has become a well-accepted treatment for this disorder. Video assistance affords excellent visualization of thoracic anatomy, which allows the procedure to be done quickly with few complications. However, despite the ease of performing ETS, complications can occur unless thoracic anatomy and physiology are well-understood. Awareness of possible intraoperative and postoperative complications is essential if this procedure is gong to be performed safely.

Facial blushing, associated with social phobia, may have severe negative impact on the quality of daily life. The first line of treatment should be psychological and/or pharmacologic. In severe cases not responding to nonsurgical treatment, surgical sympathetic denervation is an option. A thorough disclosure of effects, complications, and side effects is mandatory and patient selection is crucial to obtain high patient satisfaction from surgical treatment.

Primary plantar hyperhidrosis is defined as excessive secretion of the sweat glands of the feet and may lead to significant limitations in private and professional lifestyle and reduction of health-related quality of life. Conservative therapy measures usually fail to provide sufficient relieve of symptoms and do not allow long-lasting elimination of hyperhidrosis. Endoscopic lumbar sympathectomy appears to be a safe and effective procedure for eliminating excessive sweating of the feet and improves quality of life of patients with severe plantar hyperhidrosis.

# THORACIC SURGERY CLINICS

**RELATED INTEREST**

*Dermatologic Clinics,* Volume 32, Issue 4 (October 2014)
**Hyperhidrosis**
David M. Pariser, *Editor*
Available at: www.derm.theclinics.com

**THE CLINICS ARE AVAILABLE ONLINE!**
Access your subscription at:
www.theclinics.com

# Preface
# Hyperhidrosis

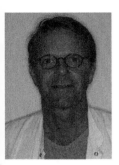

Peter B. Licht, MD, PhD
*Editor*

Millions of patients worldwide still suffer from primary hyperhidrosis, and with increasing awareness and access to the Internet, it is likely that more patients will seek treatment.

The literature on surgical management of primary hyperhidrosis had increased tremendously over the last two decades, and this is the second issue of *Thoracic Surgery Clinics* devoted to hyperhidrosis.

We begin with historical perspectives that acknowledge our sympathetic surgical heritage and bring us up to present time. Then, we move to mechanisms of pathophysiology, which are getting clearer, although we still don't have a deeper understanding why some patients develop primary hyperhidrosis. The vast majority, however, are adequately treated by nonsurgical methods that are constantly improving and will likely reduce the need for surgery in the future. The latest developments are consequently reviewed in detail.

Any professional involved in diagnosis and management of patients with hyperhidrosis will likely recognize that despite nonsurgical treatments some patients remain so disabled that they ask for sympathetic surgery despite a high risk of side effects. The key to success when medical treatment fails therefore lies in meticulous patient selection, which is discussed in a separate article.

Even when the indication for surgery has been established, there is still disagreement and conflicting opinions concerning which surgical procedure is better for primary hyperhidrosis. More than 1000 papers have been published, predominately nonrandomized studies, and it is apparent that there is little consensus about level and extent of targeting the sympathetic chain. An evidence-based review therefore brings us up-to-date with the literature.

One of the most controversial topics in sympathetic surgery is which surgical technique is better: resection, transection, ablation or clipping, which is claimed to a reversible procedure. Whether clipping is truly reversible is hotly debated, but data are accumulated and reviewed in an up-to-date overview, including possible mechanisms of reversibility. It is only fair to say that sympathetic surgeons should switch to clipping if it is truly reversible, and conversely, they should abandon clipping if it is not, because some patients are likely to accept sympathetic surgery under false premises if they are told that the operation is reversible.

Despite thorough information and meticulous patient selection, some patients still regret sympathetic surgery because of side effects. Severe compensatory sweating is the most frequent cause, but less common side effects are also reviewed in this issue. Quality-of-life investigations following sympathetic surgery have emerged in the literature and are reviewed, just as newer pharmacological treatments of compensatory sweating are presented in separate articles. A newer surgical option to treat patients who regret surgery is the promising reversal procedure by robotic technology.

Finally, facial blushing and plantar hyperhidrosis are rare but growing indications for sympathetic surgery that are discussed separately.

From the list of expert authors in this issue of *Thoracic Surgery Clinics*, it is apparent that sympathetic surgery is not only done by thoracic surgeons. Instead, these procedures are performed

Thorac Surg Clin 26 (2016) ix–x
http://dx.doi.org/10.1016/j.thorsurg.2016.08.010
1547-4127/16/© 2016 Published by Elsevier Inc.

by dedicated surgeons across surgical subspecialties, who are interested in primary hyperhidrosis and all its complexity. For years, many of these surgeons have met at the biannual meeting for the International Society of Sympathetic Surgery, joining forces to promote better research, which is desperately needed in this field.

I am indebted to the Consulting Editor, M. Blair Marshall, for giving me the opportunity to act as Guest Editor, and to the staff at Elsevier, in particular, Susan Showalter, for their kind assistance throughout this process without which this issue would not have been possible. Finally, I would like to thank all the authors who participated in this project. I am convinced that their outstanding contributions will provide the readers with an up-to-date overview of this interesting and complex topic.

Peter B. Licht, MD, PhD
Department of Cardiothoracic Surgery
Odense University Hospital
29 Søndre Boulevard
Odense, Denmark DK-5000

E-mail address:
peter.licht@rsyd.dk

# The History of Sympathetic Surgery

Moshe Hashmonai, MD, FACS

## KEYWORDS

- Sympathetic surgery • Hyperhidrosis • Sympathetic anatomy • Sympathetic physiology • History

## KEY POINTS

- The history of how the anatomy and physiology of the sympathetic system was elucidated is reported.
- The evolution of indications for which sympathetic ablation has been performed is stated.
- The methods of sympathetic surgery are described.
- The last step of sympathetic surgery, the endoscopic approach, is reported in detail.

## ANATOMY AND FUNCTION

The existence of an autonomic nervous system has been known since antiquity. Galen was the first physician to describe the system.[1] However, his description was erroneous, because it reported a common vagosympathetic trunk. Unlike some others, this mistake was repeated by Vesalius[2] in 1555. Eustachius was the first to report the separation of the vagus from the sympathetic trunk in his posthumous publication of 1744.[1] In the same period, a first step in understanding the physiology of the sympathetic system was made by du Petit who reported in 1727 that cervical sympathetic ablation resulted in miosis.[3] By the end of the eighteenth century, the anatomy of the sympathetic nervous system was fairly well described, unlike the comprehension of its function. It was Claude Bernard[3] who supplied the first major physiologic understanding of the system in 1852. He observed that section of the cervical sympathetic system involved ptosis and enophthalmos as well, and produced peripheral vasodilatation. He also proved that galvanic stimulation of the system resulted in the opposite phenomena. An additional advance in elucidating the physiology of the sympathetic system was made by Gaskell,[4] who reported that section of the sympathetic supply to the lower limb muscle temporarily increased the venous return from the muscles, and increased the temperature. In his comprehensive subsequent publication,[5] the basic anatomic and physiologic concepts of the autonomic (involuntary, as it was called at the time) nervous system were established.

Some further observations were made by Woollard and Norrish,[6] who specified the regional distribution of the system. An additional important anatomic feature was reported by Kuntz,[7] who described sympathetic vertical postganglionic filaments in the upper chest, bypassing the ganglia, to which he attributed incomplete sympathetic denervation of the upper limb following stellate ganglionectomy.[8] In addition, concerning the sympathetic supply of the hand, the importance of the second thoracic spinal segment in the preganglionic sympathetic innervation was emphasized by Atlas,[9] whereas Goetz and Marr[10] outlined the importance of the second thoracic ganglion for the sympathetic supply of the upper extremity. The beginning of sympathetic surgery was based on the initial anatomic and physiologic knowledge (and early misconceptions) accumulated by the end of the nineteenth century.

Disclosure: The author has nothing to disclose.
Department of Surgery, Rambam Medical Center & Faculty of Medicine, Technion – Israel Institute of Technology, PO Box 359, Zikhron Ya'akov, Haifa 3095202, Israel
E-mail address: hasmonai@inter.net.il

Thorac Surg Clin 26 (2016) 383–388
http://dx.doi.org/10.1016/j.thorsurg.2016.06.001
1547-4127/16/© 2016 Elsevier Inc. All rights reserved.

thoracic.theclinics.com

## OPERATIONS AND INDICATIONS

The first clinical surgical sympathectomy was performed at the level of the neck by Alexander[11] in 1889 and was intended for the treatment of epilepsy. Ionescu[12] and Jaboulay[13] performed the same operation to treat exophthalmos in 1896. It was Jaboulay[14] as well who, in 1899, performed the first sympathetic operation (periarterial denudation) for ischemic lesions. In the same year, François-Franck[15] extended the list of indications reporting cervical sympathectomies for glaucoma and what he termed "idiotie." Following the work of Jaboulay, Leriche[16] emphasized the use of sympathetic surgery for the healing of ischemic ulcers.[17] A new indication for sympathetic ablation was introduced by Kotzareff[18] in 1920, who performed the first sympathectomy for hyperhidrosis. In the same year, Ionescu[19] published the use of sympathetic ablation for the treatment of angina pectoris. Brüning[20] extended its application to Raynaud phenomenon and scleroderma. The first lumbar sympathectomy was performed by Royle[21] on September 1, 1923 for spastic paralysis. The same operation was performed for ischemic lesions of the lower limb by Diez[22] in Buenos Aires in 1924.

Following these pioneering operations, sympathetic ablation became a well-established procedure and a multitude of indications were added, whereas some of the early ones became obsolete. A systematic review of past and present indications for sympathetic ablation was published recently.[23]

## METHODS OF SYMPATHETIC ABLATION

The early sympathetic ablations were performed by resecting the cervical ganglia, inevitably resulting in Horner syndrome. Jaboulay[14] was the first to attempt perivascular denudation to obtain sympathetic ablation. Although largely adopted and practiced by Leriche,[16] the results of this technique were considered insufficient. Diez[22] improved the technique by dissecting the major nerves of the extremities (median and sciatic), the so-called nervous fascicular dissociation. Further improvement was obtained by the addition of sympathetic ganglionectomy. Concerning the lower limb, following a visit of William Mayo to Sydney, where he saw Royle operating, on return to the Mayo Clinic he incited his neurosurgeon colleague, Adson, to perform a sympathetic ablation for spastic paralysis.[1] In the same clinic, Brown, a physician with an interest in vascular medicine, incited Adson to perform the operation for ischemia.[1] The first operations combined ganglionectomy and iliac periarterial stripping,[24] but later Adson restricted his procedure to ganglionectomy.[25] Encouraged by his success, Adson applied the procedure to the upper limb, and developed the posterior approach to ablate the sympathetic chain.[26] His method was modified by White and colleagues[27] and later again by Smithwick,[28] who adjoined transection of the anterior and posterior roots to the ganglionectomy (section of the intercostal nerves at the junction of the roots). However, the posterior approach is mutilating, requiring removal of paravertebral rib sections, and involves a difficult convalescence. To circumvent these drawbacks, Telford[29,30] developed the supraclavicular approach. This approach entails a fairly painless postoperative course. However, the proximity of several important nerves and vessels during access made the operation technically demanding, which led to the development of 2 additional techniques, both involving open access of the pleural cavity. First described by Goetz and Marr,[10] and later by Palumbo,[31] the anterior approach never gained popularity. In contrast, the transaxillary approach described by Atkins[32] achieved a wide popularity and was adopted by many surgeons, whereas the posterior-dorsal access was abandoned.

In 1942, Hughes[33] reported the thoracoscopic approach for sympathectomy. In 1939 he performed 5 splanchnicectomies by this approach. Independently in 1944, Goetz and Marr[10] described the use of thoracoscopy for the ablation of the second thoracic ganglion. Kux E[34] adopted this approach and in 1951 published a multitude of thoracoscopic sympathectomies and vagotomies for duodenal ulcers, hypertension, angina, and diabetes. Twenty seven years later, Kux M[35] published the first large series of endoscopic sympathectomies performed for hyperhidrosis. With the advent of videoendoscopy in daily surgical practice, the open technique became obsolete. However, a recently published case represents a warning that an open approach may still be required.[36]

During the first operations, 2 ports were used.[10,33] Kux M[35] used a single port through which the videoscope and operating instrument were introduced simultaneously. The use of 1 port was suitable for sympathetic electroablation. For surgeons who persisted in excising the ganglia, a 3-port technique was initially used.[37] Later, the same investigators managed to excise the ganglia using 1 port for the operating instruments and 1 for the scope.[38] Drott and Claes[39] reported the first large series of upper dorsal sympathetic ablations, using a single port through which they ablated the appropriate section of the chain with diathermy.

In 1992, these 2 investigators organized, in Borås, Sweden, the first international symposium on sympathetic surgery and in 2000, together with the author, were the founders of the International Society of Sympathetic Surgery.

The fate of the open lumbar sympathectomy was similar to that of thoracic sympathectomy. It was supplanted by the endoscopic method. The intraperitoneal access was first reported in humans by Soderstrom[40] in 1975. After an initial animal study,[41] the retroperitoneal approach was applied to humans and became the standard for lumbar sympathectomies.[42]

## THE EFFECT OF THE THORACOSCOPIC APPROACH ON SYMPATHETIC SURGERY

The advent of thoracoscopy revolutionized sympathetic surgery in several ways.

### Methods of Ablation

During the era of open surgery, resection of the appropriate sympathetic ganglia was the golden standard. With the advent of thoracoscopy, cauterizing the ganglion and/or transecting the chain using scissors, diathermy, clips,[43] or harmonic scalpel[44] supplanted excision because resecting the ganglia during thoracoscopy requires a much more advanced surgical skill. However, a review comparing resection of the ganglia versus ablation delineated the difference in results: invariably dry hands in the former and a substantial percentage of failures and recurrences in the latter.[45]

### Level and Extent of Ablation

During the era of open surgery, excision of the second thoracic ganglion was considered imperative to obtain sympathetic denervation of the hand. In addition, not only the second ganglion but the third and often the first ganglia were excised as well. During the same period, results were categorized either as dry hands (success) or persistent perspiration (failure). The occurrence of compensatory hyperhidrosis (CHH) was reported, but never seemed to be an issue in the literature.[46] With the advent of endoscopy, totally anhidrotic hands started to be considered as palmar overdryness and were judged by some investigators to be an undesired result of sympathectomy.[47] Instead of simply dry or wet, a range of reduced degrees of perspiration was introduced, raising the question of what degree is desirable and how to obtain it. It seems that lowering the level of ablation by mistake and obtaining apparently satisfactory results prompted surgeons to deviate from the axiom that $G_2 \pm G_1 \pm G_3$ (G - sympathetic ganglion) resection is required to abolish palmar hyperhidrosis.[48] Reducing the extent of ablation to a single ganglion, lowering the level of ablation, and ablating the sympathetic system by methods other than resection were adopted. However, an extensive review of the literature,[49] which found 42 techniques of sympathetic ablation, did not support the claims that lowering the level of ablation, using a method of ablation other than resection, or restricting the extent of sympathetic ablation for primary palmar hyperhidrosis results in less CHH. Although Cerfolio and colleagues[50] advised restricting and lowering the level of ablation in order to reduce CHH, another recent controlled trial[51] did not support that lowering the level of sympathetic ablation affected the incidence or severity of this sequela. Limiting the extent of ablation to reduce CHH was not supported by 2 other studies. In one, limiting $T_2$-$T_3$ to $T_2$-only sympathetic ablation did not reduce the amount of CHH.[52] Similar results were obtained comparing $T_2$-$T_3$ down to $T_2$-$T_6$ resections.[53] Controversy persists.

### Techniques of Access

Thoracoscopy is performed by penetrating the pleural cavity through the intercostal spaces in the chest wall. Numerous sites have been used, and 2 variations were recently suggested. The first is the use of a single port, inserted transumbilically.[54] It entails violation of the peritoneum, perforation of both diaphragms, and requires special instrumentation. The advantages of having a single camouflaged scar in the umbilicus versus these drawbacks has been questioned.[55] However, the instigators of this technique have been using it in humans[56] with apparent success.[57]

A second access was examined by the NOTES (natural orifice translumenal endoscopic surgery) principle in an animal study using the transesophageal route.[58] The investigators succeeded in performing a bilateral thoracic sympathetic ablation by this technique, proving the feasibility of the method. However, it is doubtful that perforating the esophagus and violating the sterility of the mediastinum can be justified solely to avoid 2 small scars on each side of the chest. Feasibility is not equivalent to desirability!

In addition, robotics have been used in sympathetic surgery, and a series of thoracoscopic sympathetic ablations performed with robotic instrumentation has been published.[59] This method provides a three-dimensional view during surgery. It remains to be proved whether this advantage, at the cost of doubling the number of portholes and the 4-fold increase in operating time and hospital stay, outweighs the two-dimensional view provided by the standard instrumentation.

## SUMMARY

Since the first clinical sympathectomy, performed in 1889, sympathetic surgery has substantially evolved. Early indications have become obsolete, as has ischemia caused by arterial occlusion, which was the major indication for sympathetic surgery for many decades.

At present, primary hyperhidrosis is the main indication for sympathectomy. Several other indications are still valid, but are rarely used. Thoracoscopy supplanted the 4 open approaches and endoscopy (either transperitoneal or retroperitoneal) replaced laparotomy. For upper thoracic sympathetic ablation, excision of the second thoracic ganglion alone or with the first and/or third ganglia was the standard during the open surgery era. With the advent of thoracoscopy, a plethora of modifications related to the level, extent, and type of ablation were proposed in order to attenuate CHH. It is possible that lowering the level, reducing the extent, and transecting the chain instead of excising/thermoablating the ganglia would result in attenuating CHH, but this achievement is at the expense of reaching a lesser degree of sweat reduction and a higher percentage of recurrences. The ideal operation for hyperhidrosis of the face and upper limbs remains to be defined. To do so, controlled double-blind studies with quantitative measurements of sweat production are required.

## REFERENCES

1. Royle JP. A history of sympathectomy. Aust N Z J Surg 1999;69:302–7.
2. Vesalius A. The fabric of the human body. In: Garrison DH, Hast MH, editors. An annotated translation of the 1543 and 1955 editions of "De Humanis Corporis Fabrica". Basel (Switzerland): Karger; 2014. p. 845 (corresponding to p. 512 of the 1555 original edition).
3. Bernard C. Sur les effets de la section de la portion céphalique du grand sympathique. C R Seances Soc Biol Fil 1852;4:168–70.
4. Gaskell WH. Further researches on the vasomotor nerves of ordinary muscles. J Physiol 1879;1: 262–426.15.
5. Gaskell WH. The involuntary nervous system. London: Longmans; Green & Co; 1916.
6. Woollard HH, Norrish RE. The anatomy of the peripheral sympathetic nervous system. Br J Surg 1933; 21:83–103.
7. Kuntz A. Distribution of the sympathetic rami to the brachial plexus: its relation to sympathectomy affecting the upper extremity. Arch Surg 1927;15: 871–7.
8. Kuntz A, Alexander WF, Furcolo CL. Complete sympathetic denervation of the upper limb. Ann Surg 1938;107:25–31.
9. Atlas LN. The role of the second thoracic spinal segment in the preganglionic sympathetic innervation of the human hand – surgical implications. Ann Surg 1941;114:456–61.
10. Goetz RH, Marr JAS. The importance of the second thoracic ganglion for the sympathetic supply of the upper extremities. Clin Proc 1944;3:102–14.
11. Alexander W. The treatment of epilepsy. Edinburgh (United Kingdom): YJ Pentland; 1889. p. 27–106.
12. Ionescu T. Resecția totală și bilaterală a simpaticului cervicul în cazuri de epilepsie și gușă exoftalmică. Romania Med 1896;4:479–91.
13. Jaboulay M. Chirurgie du grand sympathique et du corps thyroïde (Les différents goîtres). Articles originaux et observations réunis et publiés par le Dr. Etienne Martin. Lyon (France): A Stock & Cie; 1900. p. 3–5.
14. Jaboulay M. Le traitement de quelques troubles trophiques du pied et de la jambe par la dénudation de l'artère fémorale et la distension des nerfs vasculaires. Lyon Med 1899;91:467–8.
15. François-Franck M. Signification physiologique de la résection du sympathique dans la maladies de Basedow, l'épilepsie, l'idiotie et le glaucome. Bull Acad Méd 1899;41:565–94.
16. Leriche R. De l'élongation et de la section des nerfs périvasculaires dans certains syndromes douloureux d'origine artérielle et dans quelques troubles trophiques. Lyon Chir 1913;10:378–82.
17. Leriche R. Some researches on the periarterial sympathetics. Ann Surg 1921;74:385–93.
18. Kotzareff A. Résection partielle du tronc sympathique cervical droit pour hyperhidrose unilatérale. Rev Med Suisse Romande 1920;40:111–3.
19. Ionescu T. Angine the poitrine guérie par la résection du sympathique cervicothoracique. Bull Acad Méd Paris 1920;84:93–102.
20. Brüning F. Zur Technik der kombinierten Resektionsmethode sämtlicher sympathischen Nervenbahnen am Halse. Zentralbl Chir 1923;5:1056–9.
21. Royle ND. A new operative procedure in the treatment of spastic paralysis and its experimental basis. Med J Aust 1924;1:77–86.
22. Diez J. Un nuevo método de simpatectomia perifèrica para el tratamiento de las afecciones tròficas y gangrenosas de los miembros. Bol Trab Soc Cir B Aires 1924;8:792–806.
23. Hashmonai M, Cameron AEP, Licht PB, et al. Thoracic sympathectomy: a review of current indications. Surg Endosc 2016;30(4):1255–69.
24. Adson AW, Brown GE. Treatment of Raynaud's disease by lumbar ramisectomy and ganglionectomy

and perivascular sympathetic neurectomy of the common iliacs. JAMA 1925;84:1908–10.

25. Adson AW, Brown GE. The treatment of Raynaud's disease by resection of the upper thoracic and lumbar sympathetic ganglia and trunks. Surg Gynecol Obstet 1929;48:577–603.

26. Adson AW, Brown GE. Raynaud's disease of the upper extremities: successful treatment by resection of the sympathetic cervicothoracic and second thoracic ganglions and the intervening trunk. JAMA 1929;92:444–9.

27. White JC, Smithwick RH, Allen AW, et al. A new muscle splitting incision for resection of the upper thoracic sympathetic ganglia. Surg Gynecol Obstet 1933;56:651–7.

28. Smithwick RH. Modified dorsal sympathectomy for vascular spasm (Raynaud's disease) of the upper extremity. Ann Surg 1936;104:339–50.

29. Telford ED. The technique of sympathectomy. Br J Surg 1935;23:448–50.

30. Telford ED. Sympathetic denervation of the upper extremity. Lancet 1938;1:70–2.

31. Palumbo LT. Anterior transthoracic approach for upper thoracic sympathectomy. Arch Surg 1956;72:659–66.

32. Atkins HJB. Sympathectomy by the axillary approach. Lancet 1954;266:538–9.

33. Hughes J. Endothoracic sympathectomy. Proc R Soc Med 1942;35:585–6.

34. Kux E. The endoscopic approach to the vegetative nervous system and its therapeutic possibilities. Chest J 1951;20:139–47.

35. Kux M. Thoracic endoscopic sympathectomy in palmar and axillary hyperhidrosis. Arch Surg 1978;113:264–6.

36. Spolyanski G, Hashmonai M, Rudin M, et al. Video-assisted open supraclavicular sympathectomy following air embolism. JSLS 2012;16:337–9.

37. Hashmonai M, Kopelman D, Schein M. Thoracoscopic versus open supraclavicular upper dorsal sympathectomy. A prospective randomized trial. Eur J Surg 1994;160(Suppl 572):13–6.

38. Kopelman D, Hashmonai M, Ehrenreich M, et al. Upper dorsal thoracoscopic sympathectomy for palmar hyperhidrosis: improved intermediate-term results. J Vasc Surg 1996;24:194–9.

39. Drott C, Claes G. Hyperhidrosis treated by thoracoscopic sympathectomy. Cardiovasc Surg 1996;4:788–90.

40. Soderstrom RM. Unusual uses of laparoscopy. J Reprod Med 1975;15:77–8.

41. Bannenberg JJ, Hourlay P, Meijer DW, et al. Retroperitoneal endoscopic lumbar sympathectomy: laboratory and clinical experience. Endosc Surg Allied Technol 1995;3:16–20.

42. Hourlay P, Vangertruyden G, Verduyckt F, et al. Endoscopic extraperitoneal lumbar sympathectomy. Surg Endosc 1995;9:530–3.

43. Lin C-C, Mo L-R, Lee L-S, et al. Thoracoscopic $T_2$-sympathetic block by clipping – a better and reversible operation for treatment of hyperhidrosis palmaris: experience with 326 cases. Eur J Surg 1998;164(Suppl 580):13–6.

44. Kopelman D, Bahous H, Assalia A, et al. Upper dorsal thoracoscopic sympathectomy for palmar hyperhidrosis. The use of harmonic scalpel versus diathermy. Ann Chir Gynaecol 2001;90:203–5.

45. Hashmonai M, Assalia A, Kopelman D. Thoracoscopic sympathectomy for palmar hyperhidrosis. Ablate or resect? Surg Endosc 2001;15:435–41.

46. Adar R, Kurchin A, Zweig A, et al. Palmar hyperhidrosis and its surgical treatment: a report of 100 cases. Ann Surg 1977;186:34–41.

47. Chang Y-T, Li H-P, Lee J-Y, et al. Treatment of palmar hyperhidrosis: $T_4$ level compared with $T_3$ and $T_2$. Ann Surg 2007;246:330–6.

48. Lin C-C, Wu H-H. Endoscopic $T_4$-sympathetic block by clamping ($ESB_4$) in treatment of hyperhidrosis palmaris et axillaris – experiences of 165 cases. Ann Chir Gynaecol 2001;90:167–9.

49. Kopelman D, Hashmonai M. The correlation between the method of sympathetic ablation for palmar hyperhidrosis and the occurrence of compensatory hyperhidrosis: a review. World J Surg 2008;32:2343–56.

50. Cerfolio RJ, de Campos JRM, Bryant AS, et al. The Society of Thoracic Surgeons expert consensus for the surgical treatment of hyperhidrosis. Ann Thorac Surg 2011;91:1642–8.

51. Cai S, Huang S, An J, et al. Effect of lowering or restricting sympathectomy levels on compensatory sweating. Clin Auton Res 2014;24:143–9.

52. Licht PB, Pilegaard HK. Severity of compensatory sweating after thoracoscopic sympathectomy. Ann Thorac Surg 2004;78:427–31.

53. Gunn BM, Davis DM, Speicher JE, et al. Expended level of sympathetic chain removal does not increase the incidence or severity of compensatory hyperhidrosis after endoscopic thoracic sympathectomy. J Thorac Cardiovasc Surg 2014;148:2673–6.

54. Zhu L-H, Chen L, Yang S, et al. Embryonic NOTES thoracic sympathectomy for palmar hyperhidrosis: results of a novel technique and comparison with the conventional VATS procedure. Surg Endosc 2013;27:4124–9.

55. Hashmonai M, Licht PB, Schick CH, et al. Transumbilical thoracic sympathectomy with an ultrathin flexible endoscope in a series of 38 patients. Surg Endosc 2014;28:1380–1 [Letter to the Editor].

56. Zhu L-H, Wand W, Yang S, et al. Transumbilical thoracic sympathectomy with an ultrathin flexible endoscope in a series of 38 patients. Surg Endosc 2013;27:2149–55.

57. Zhu L-H, Du Q, Chen L, et al. One-year follow-up period after transumbilical thoracic sympathectomy for hyperhidrosis: outcomes and consequences. J Thorac Cardiovasc Surg 2014;147:25–9.

58. Turner BG, Gee DW, Cizginer S, et al. Feasibility of endoscopic transesophageal thoracic sympathectomy (with video). Gastrointest Endosc 2010;71:171–5.

59. Coveliers H, Meyer M, Gharagozloo F, et al. Robotic selective postganglionic thoracic sympathectomy for the treatment of hyperhidrosis. Ann Thorac Surg 2013;95:269–74.

# Pathophysiology of Hyperhidrosis

Christoph H. Schick, PD Dr*

## KEYWORDS

- Hyperhidrosis • Pathophysiology • Thermal regulation • Diagnostics

## KEY POINTS

- For many surgeons, hyperhidrosis is still a disease of unknown origin.
- As a neurologic disorder of the autonomic nervous system, it is mandatory for surgeons to know about the fundamental relationship between thermoregulation, hyperhidrosis, and pathophysiology.
- Knowledge about physiology, anatomic pathways, and diagnostic procedures helps sympathetic surgeons to find the best treatment for their patients.

Studies and case reports on excessive sweating frequently state that hyperhidrosis is a disease whose origin and mechanism are unknown. However, the term excessive is rarely based on systematic diagnostic measurements, instead being a description of the symptoms from patient histories. The term excessive leads to the impression that hyperhidrosis is purely a problem involving the quantity of sweat, whereas it is a change in the control mechanism of sweating in which the need for and production of sweat are strongly disproportionate. This lack of proportion is perceived by those affected to be a limitation of activities of daily living and is thus pathologic.

## THERMAL REGULATION

Sweat is produced by the eccrine and apocrine glands in the skin. The existence of mixed forms has not been verified. Apocrine sweat glands become active after the onset of puberty and release pheromones and other substances into the infundibular portion of the hair follicle, which are converted to odors by sebum and bacteria. Eccrine glands constitute most of the sweat glands and are mainly responsible for thermal regulation. They produce a thin, hypotonic secretion. They develop during the embryonic stage; no new glands are formed after birth.[1,2] The eccrine sweat glands are distributed unevenly over the body, with the greatest density in the axillary, palmar, and plantar regions.[3]

In addition to generating heat as a reaction to external cold, thermal regulation mainly involves dissipation of body heat. Body heat builds up because of an increased metabolic rate, muscle activity, dietary-induced thermogenesis, and environmental effects such as increased ambient temperature or thermal radiation. The body dissipates heat through radiation, conduction, convection, and evaporation. Although heat loss from radiation is around 10%, the percentage from conduction and convection is around 35%. Ambient conditions such as clothing and airflow have a great effect. Evaporation is the most effective method of heat dissipation; 1 L of evaporated liquid removes 580 kcal of heat from the body. As the ambient temperature increases, energy transfer by radiation, conduction, and convection becomes less significant and evaporation of sweat and water

Conflicts of Interest: None.
Department of Surgery, University of Erlangen-Nuremberg, Erlangen, Germany
* Deutsches Hyperhidrosezentrum DHHZ, German Hyperhidrosis Center, St.-Bonifatius-Street 5, Munich D-81541, Germany.
E-mail address: schick@dhhz.de

Thorac Surg Clin 26 (2016) 389–393
http://dx.doi.org/10.1016/j.thorsurg.2016.06.002
1547-4127/16/© 2016 Elsevier Inc. All rights reserved.

from the respiratory tract are the only effective mechanisms. A significant concomitant factor is the relative humidity. If the relative humidity is high, the ambient water vapor pressure approaches that of moist skin and evaporation is hindered.

A rapid onset of sweating is important because even small increases in body temperature can lead to reduced performance. In sports, this has led to the respective recommendations from the International Olympic Committee and Fédération Internationale de Football Association regarding behavior and cooling-down phases.[4,5]

## HYPERHIDROSIS

The purpose of sweating is to restore the body's normal temperature or maintain the balance between heat input and dissipation.[6] Ideally, heating and cooling the body should be proportionate to each other. This kind of sweating is considered normal even when it is increased; for example, when the ambient temperature is high. In individuals affected by hyperhidrosis, the sweating reaction is much more pronounced and does not occur in proportion. The exponential increase in sweating leads to the formation of droplets on the skin that may even drip off. However, sweat that drips off is lost to the cooling function and is therefore not useful. Those affected by hyperhidrosis do not become aware of their excessive sweating until water drops form and run off their skin and their clothing becomes damp. This experience is perceived to be unpleasant and the emotional reaction exacerbates the effect.

To facilitate the differentiation from diseases in which sweat attacks are among the symptoms, it is customary to classify hyperhidrosis into secondary and primary forms.[7] Secondary hyperhidrosis occurs less frequently than primary and is the result of an underlying disease. Secondary hyperhidrosis can also occur in circumscribed areas caused by autonomic degenerative disorders, cerebral infarction, spinal cord injury, gustatory sweating, and Harlequin syndrome, and is associated with other disorders of the central and peripheral nervous systems. Secondary hyperhidrosis is frequently a generalized occurrence associated with disorders of the central and peripheral nervous systems, in conjunction with fever and infections, caused by metabolic and systemic diseases, malignant diseases, and poisoning, and also induced by drugs.

Primary hyperhidrosis is the most common disorder of the sweat function[8] and occurs primarily in the armpits, hands, and feet; craniofacial and generalized sweating are less common. There is

little information about the prevalence. Around 0.6% to 2.8% of the population is affected.[9,10] Both genders are affected equally, with the onset of the symptoms usually before age 25 years. It may occur in phases or continuously, but usually not at night. Primary hyperhidrosis is induced by thermal triggers, physical activity, and emotional stress, and occurs (especially when triggered by emotional stress) regardless of the ambient temperature. Emotional sweating is often ascribed the function of a feedback signal for highly emotional sensory, cognitive, and behavioral processes.[11] In addition, it gives the hands and feet a better grip. Emotion-induced sweating is regulated by the neocortical and limbic centers.[12–14] The spinal and peripheral pathways are the same as with thermoregulatory sweating,[15] in which mostly sweat glands on the palms, soles of the feet, armpits, and face are triggered.[6] Simultaneously, emotion-induced vasoconstrictors are activated, leading to cold hands and feet, whereas thermoregulatory sweating causes vasodilatation.[16] However, thermoregulatory and emotional sweating cannot be separated[17] and mutually affect each other.[15]

## DIAGNOSING HYPERHIDROSIS

The quantitative static analysis of sweat is performed using gravimetry by collecting sweat on previously weighed filter paper at representative sites of the body for a specified period. The difference in weight is equivalent to the quantity of sweat in milligrams per unit time.[18] This method is suitable for the armpits, hands, and feet. There are no clear standard amounts. A quantity of greater than 50 mg/min in the armpits and greater than 20 mg/min on the hands is considered to be pathologic.[19]

Sweating can be measured over time using dynamic quantitative sudometry.[20,21] Dried gas is run through a measuring chamber placed on the hand and the quantity of moisture absorbed from the surface of the skin is measured. Sweating can be measured at baseline, after thermal provocation, and after stimulation; for example, by iontophoresis of acetylcholine (quantitative sudomotor axon reflex test).[22]

The Minor starch-iodine test is a semiquantitative test[23] that is used in circumscribed areas in the armpits, hands, feet, and head, but can also be used for whole-body mapping. The sweat distribution pattern allows conclusions to be drawn about the cause of the sweat disorder.[24]

The most important diagnostic tool is the patient history. As qualitative criteria, the onset of symptoms in childhood or adolescence; uncontrollable, non–temperature-related, sweating (sweating in winter); symmetric pattern; absence of sweating during the night; and familial disposition suggest hyperhidrosis. The most important criterion has proved to be the Hyperhidrosis Disease Severity Scale,[25] which classifies sweating in 4 categories: never noticeable and never interfering with daily activities, tolerable but sometimes interfering, barely tolerable and frequently interfering, and intolerable and always interfering. This easily understandable scale indicates serious hyperhidrosis requiring treatment at a score of 3 or 4.

## PATHOPHYSIOLOGY OF HYPERHIDROSIS

The physiology of sweating has been thoroughly discussed in the literature[26] and the central and peripheral mechanisms have been described.[11] Sweating is regulated in the autonomic nervous system via the sympathetic nervous system and, in warm-blooded animals, its cooling function keeps the body temperature constant. Thermal receptors are distributed throughout the body: in the skin, the internal organs, the brain stem,[27] the spinal cord,[28] and in the hypothalamus[13,29] as the central regulating unit of the autonomic system. The signals reach the hypothalamus through afferent nerve fibers via the lateral spinal cord and are compared with a set value. This set value is not constant[30,31] and, depending on acclimatization processes, serves to balance increase and loss of heat.

The relationship of sudomotor dermatomes is less precise than the sensory; that is, the individual dermatomes receive sudomotor innervation from several adjacent segment levels, which is one reason why minimizing surgical sympathetic nerve blocks has results that are equally as good as extensive resections of the sympathetic trunk. The sympathetic nerve fibers coming from the thoracic spinal cord first pass through the thoracic sympathetic ganglia. The body is innervated by the efferent sudomotor fibers coming approximately from the ipsilateral segments T1 to T4 for the head, with a maximum from T2 and T3; from T2 to T5 for the hand, with a maximum from T3 and T4; from T3 to T6 for the armpits, with a maximum from T4; from T4 to T12 for the trunk; and from T10 to L4 for the leg and foot.

Innervation of the eccrine sweat glands is effected from the hypothalamus as the integration center for all thermosensory afferences[13,29] in crossed and uncrossed fibers through the pons and medulla to the spinal cord. Most fibers undergo synaptic switching on the way to the skin. This switching generally takes place in the paravertebral sympathetic ganglia, from where the sweat glands are reached postsynaptically via cholinergic fibers. The released peripheral neurotransmitter is acetylcholine, which binds to postsynaptic muscarinic receptors of the eccrine sweat glands and triggers sweating.[32]

Humans are assumed to have around 5000 preganglionic neurons per segment, with a reduction of 5% to 7% per decade.[33] This reduction may explain the frequently observed reduced sweating in the elderly and the effect described by patients of a reduction of symptoms in old age in family members who were previously more strongly affected.

The familial clustering of hyperhidrosis suggests a strong hereditary component. This hereditary component has already been mathematically confirmed in studies[34,35] and the gene locus was also determined.[36] Different loci suggest genetic heterogenicity.[37]

Hyperhidrosis is not an increase of the absolute quantity of sweat but a change in the kinetics, and thus regulation, of sweating. Small triggers lead to disproportionately strong sweating. However, there is no dysfunction of the end organ, the sweat gland. In histopathologic examinations, sweat glands of individuals affected by hyperhidrosis do not show any microscopic or macroscopic abnormalities.[38,39]

The sudomotor function can be greatly changed by disorders in the autonomic nervous system.[40] These changes can be seen in test setups in the form of a changed reflexive sweating response to triggers of sweating. Sweating disorders have been described and quantified using thermoregulatory sweat tests and quantitative sudomotor axon reflex tests.

In tests such as these, primary hyperhidrosis showed dysregulation consistent with other autonomic disorders, including sudomotor, baroreceptor, and vasomotor disorders.[41] This finding was also proved in our own studies.[42,43] The reverse correlation also applies: other autonomic disorders are also associated with changes of the sweating function.[44] In a case study, the dislocation of a brain stimulation probe for treatment of essential tremor led to hyperhidrosis caused by unintended stimulation of the hypothalamus.[45] A reduction in the inhibition of sympathetic neurons caused by trauma or stroke with damage to the insula, the hypothalamus, or the brain stem also leads to hyperhidrosis of the contralateral side; the extent of the damage correlates with the severity of hyperhidrosis.[46–48] Surgical sympathetic blocks always lead to a change in sweating in the torso,[49] which is generally termed compensatory sweating. This postoperative hyperhidrosis has only a slight compensatory effect through reducing cooling of the body surface. This effect can be better explained as a disruption of inhibition loops, similar to that from neuronal cerebral lesions. This disruption explains why the location and extent of the sympathetic block can be predictive factors for postsympathetic block sweating, as is the extent of preoperative sweating at locations not treated by the operation, especially on the trunk.

In summary, primary hyperhidrosis is a neural regulation disorder in the autonomic nervous system with pathologic hyperactivity of the sympathetic system and decoupling of hyperhidrotic regions from central thermoregulation. Affected individuals have little control of their excessive sweating, experience stress and limitations in their private and professional lives, and usually desire treatment.

## REFERENCES

1. Kuno Y. Human perspiration. Thomas CC, editor. Springfield (IL): 1956. p. 42.
2. Li HH, Zhou G, Fu XB, et al. Antigen expression of human eccrine sweat glands. J Cutan Pathol 2009; 36:318–24.
3. Sato K, Kang WH, Saga K, et al. Biology of sweat glands and their disorders. I. Normal sweat gland function. J Am Acad Dermatol 1989;20:537–63.
4. FIFA: Playing in the heat. Additional cooling breaks when WBGT is above 32°C. Available at: http://www.fifa.com/development/medical/players-health/minimising-risks/heat.html. Accessed October 4, 2013.
5. McDonagh D, Zideman D, editors. The IOC manual of emergency sports medicine. Oxford (United Kingdom): Wiley Blackwell; 2015.
6. Schondorf R. Skin potentials: normal and abnormal. In: Low PA, editor. Clinical autonomic disorders. New York: Lippincott-Raven; 1997. p. 221–31.
7. Worle B, Rapprich S, Heckmann M. Definition and treatment of primary hyperhidrosis. J Dtsch Dermatol Ges 2007;5:625–8.
8. Eisenach JH, Atkinson JL, Fealey RD. Hyperhidrosis: evolving therapies for a well-established phenomenon. Mayo Clin Proc 2005;80:657–66.
9. Adar R, Kurchin A, Zweig A, et al. Palmar hyperhidrosis and its surgical treatment: a report of 100 cases. Ann Surg 1977;186:34–41.
10. Strutton DR, Kowalski JW, Glaser DA, et al. US prevalence of hyperhidrosis and impact on individuals with axillary hyperhidrosis: results from a national survey. J Am Acad Dermatol 2004;51:241–8.
11. Schlereth T, Dieterich M, Birklein F. Hyperhidrosis – causes and treatment of enhanced sweating. Dtsch Arztebl Int 2009;106:32–7.
12. Ogawa T. Thermal influence on palmar sweating and mental influence on generalized sweating in man. Jpn J Physiol 1975;25:525–36.
13. Ogawa T, Low PA. Autonomic regulation of temperature and sweating. In: Low PA, editor. Clinical autonomic disorders. Philadelphia: Lippincott-Raven; 1997. p. 83–96.
14. Asahina M, Suzuki A, Mori M, et al. Emotional sweating response in a patient with bilateral amygdala damage. Int J Psychophysiol 2003;47:87–93.
15. Jänig W. Functions of the sympathetic innervation of the skin. In: Loewy AD, editor. Central regulation of autonomic functions. New York: Oxford University Press; 1990. p. 334–48.
16. Bini G, Hagbarth KE, Hynninen P, et al. Thermoregulatory and rhythm generating mechanisms governing the sudomotor and vasoconstrictor outflow in human cutaneous nerves. J Physiol 1980;306:537–52.
17. Sugenoya J, Ogawa T, Jmai K, et al. Cutaneous vasodilatation responses synchronize with sweat expulsions. Eur J Appl Physiol Occup Physiol 1995;71: 33–40.
18. Heckmann M, Ceballos-Baumann AO, Plewig G. Botulinum toxin A for axillary hyperhidrosis (excessive sweating). N Engl J Med 2001;344:488–93.
19. Heckmann M, Plewig G. Low-dose efficacy of botulinum toxin A for axillary hyperhidrosis: a randomized, side-by-side, open label study. Arch Dermatol 2005; 141:1255–9.
20. Low PA, Caskey PE, Tuck RR, et al. Quantitative sudomotor axon reflex test in normal and neuropathic subjects. Ann Neurol 1983;14:573–80.
21. Lang E, Foerster A, Pfannmuller D, et al. Quantitative assessment of sudomotor activity by capacitance hygrometry. Clin Auton Res 1993;3:107–15.
22. Kihara M, Opfer-Gehrking TL, Low PA. Comparison of directly stimulated with axon-reflex-mediated sudomotor responses in human subjects and in patients with diabetes. Muscle Nerve 1993;16:655–60.
23. Minor V. Ein neues Verfahren zu der klinischen Untersuchung der Schweißabsonderung. Z Neurol 1927; 101:302–8.
24. Low PA. Laboratory evaluation of autonomic function. In: Low PA, editor. Clinical autonomic disorders. Philadelphia: Lippincott-Raven; 1997. p. 179–208.
25. Solish N, Bertucci V, Dansereau A, et al. Canadian Hyperhidrosis Advisory Committee. A comprehensive approach to the recognition, diagnosis, and severity-based treatment of focal hyperhidrosis: recommendations of the Canadian Hyperhidrosis Advisory Committee. Dermatol Surg 2007;33:908–23.
26. Sato K. Clinical autonomic disorders. Boston: Little, Brown and Company; 1993.
27. Inoue S, Murakami N. Unit responses in the medulla oblongata of rabbit to changes in local and cutaneous temperature. J Physiol 1976;259:339–56.
28. Simon E. Temperature regulation: the spinal cord as a site of extrahypothalamic thermoregulatory functions. Rev Physiol Biochem Pharmacol 1974; 71:1–76.

29. Benarroch EE. Thermoregulation: recent concepts and remaining questions. Neurology 2007;69: 1293–7.

30. Nielsen M. Die Regulation der Körpertemperatur bei Muskelarbeit. Skand Arch Physiol 1938;79:193–230.

31. Glaser EM, Newling PS. The control of body temperature in thermal balance. J Physiol 1957;137:1–11.

32. Low PA, Kihara M, Cordone C. Pharmacology and morphometry of the eccrine sweat gland in vivo. In: Low PA, editor. Clinical autonomic disorders. Boston: Little, Brown and Company; 1993. p. 367–73.

33. Low PA, Okazaki H, Dyck PJ. Splanchnic preganglionic neurons in man. I. Morphometry of preganglionic cytons. Acta Neuropathol 1977;40:55–61.

34. Ro KM, Cantor RM, Lange KL, et al. Palmar hyperhidrosis: evidence of genetic transmission. J Vasc Surg 2002;35:382–6.

35. Kaufmann H, Saadia D, Polin C, et al. Primary hyperhidrosis – evidence for autosomal dominant inheritance. Clin Auton Res 2003;13:96–8.

36. Higashimoto I, Yoshiura K, Hirakawa N, et al. Primary palmar hyperhidrosis locus maps to 14q11.2-q13. Am J Med Genet A 2006;140:567–72.

37. Del Sorbo F, Brancati F, De Joanna G, et al. Primary focal hyperhidrosis in a new family not linked to known loci. Dermatology 2011;223:335–42.

38. Hurley HJ, Shelley WB. Axillary hyperhidrosis. Clinical features and local surgical management. Br J Dermatol 1966;78:127–40.

39. Bovell DL, Clunes MT, Elder HY, et al. Ultrastructure of the hyperhidrotic eccrine sweat gland. Br J Dermatol 2001;145:298–301.

40. Mathias CJ. Sympathetic nervous system disorders in man. Baillieres Clin Endocrinol Metab 1993;7: 465–90.

41. Shih CJ, Wu JJ, Lin MT. Autonomic dysfunction in palmar hyperhidrosis. J Auton Nerv Syst 1983;8: 33–43.

42. Fronek KS, Schmelz M, Krüger S, et al. Effects of gender and level of surgical sympathetic block on vasoconstrictor function. Clin Auton Res 2003; 13(Suppl 1):I74–8.

43. Schick CH, Fronek K, Held A, et al. Differential effects of surgical sympathetic block on sudomotor and vasoconstrictor function. Neurology 2003;60: 1770–6.

44. Bickel A, Axelrod FB, Marthol H, et al. Sudomotor function in familial dysautonomia. J Neurol Neurosurg Psychiatry 2004;75:275–9.

45. Diamond A, Kenney C, Almaguer M, et al. Hyperhidrosis due to deep brain stimulation in a patient with essential tremor. Case report. J Neurosurg 2007;107:1036–8.

46. Korpelainen JT, Sotaniemi KA, Myllylä VV. Asymmetric sweating in stroke: a prospective quantitative study of patients with hemispheral brain infarction. Neurology 1993;43:1211–4.

47. Rey A, Martí-Vilalta JL, Abellán MT. Contralateral hyperhidrosis secondary to the pontine infarct. Rev Neurol 1996;24:459–60.

48. Smith CD. A hypothalamic stroke producing recurrent hemihyperhidrosis. Neurology 2001;56:1394–6.

49. Schick CH, Horbach T. Sequelae of endoscopic sympathetic block. Clin Auton Res 2003; 13(Suppl 1):I36–9.

# Emerging Nonsurgical Treatments for Hyperhidrosis

Anastasia O. Kurta, DO, Dee Anna Glaser, MD*

## KEYWORDS

- Hyperhidrosis • Thermolysis • Laser • Ultrasound scan • Anticholinergic drugs • Botulinum toxin
- Iontophoresis

## KEY POINTS

- Botulinum toxin is easy to deliver and provides excellent and predictable results with minimal side effects.
- Tap water iontophoresis therapy is a cost-effective treatment modality, especially useful for palmoplantar hyperhidrosis.
- Devices delivering energy to destroy sweat glands in the axillary region provide long-lasting reduction in sweating with a good safety profile.
- Topical anticholinergic agents are being investigated and may provide efficacy with fewer systemic adverse effects.
- Despite new therapies, more research is needed to further enhance hyperhidrosis treatment.

## INTRODUCTION

Primary focal hyperhidrosis is characterized by excessive sweating greater than what is required for normal physiologic temperature regulation and that cannot be attributed to secondary medical conditions or medications. Hyperhidrosis affects approximately 3% of the global population and negatively influences quality of life and physical and emotional well-being.[1] Areas commonly affected are axillae, palms and soles, face, scalp, inframammary region, and groin. Its impact on affected individuals' quality of life is comparable to many common dermatologic disorders such as psoriasis and acne.[2] The effect of hyperhidrosis on quality of life can be assessed in multiple ways. Two commonly used measures are the Dermatology Life Quality Index and the Hyperhidrosis Disease Severity Scale (HDSS), a 4-point, validated scale that measures the severity of patients' hyperhidrosis based on how it affects daily activities (**Box 1**).[3]

A variety of treatment options exist for hyperhidrosis, some depending on the anatomic region that is affected. Therapies can include the use of:

- Botulinum toxins
- Tap water iontophoresis
- Microwave energy thermolysis
- Externally applied ultrasound
- Lasers
- Anticholinergic drugs
- Alpha-2 adrenergic agonists (such as clonidine)
- Beta blockers
- Endoscopic thoracic sympathectomy

A.O. Kurta is serving as a sub-investigator for Allergan and Ulthera. D.A. Glaser has served as advisor for Allergan, Galderma, Miramar Labs, and Unilever. She has been an investigator for Allergan, Miramar Labs, and Ulthera and received a research grant from Allergan.
Department of Dermatology, Saint Louis University School of Medicine, 1755 South Grand Boulevard, St Louis, MO 63104, USA
* Corresponding author.
E-mail address: glasermd@slu.edu

Thorac Surg Clin 26 (2016) 395–402
http://dx.doi.org/10.1016/j.thorsurg.2016.06.003
1547-4127/16/© 2016 Elsevier Inc. All rights reserved.

thoracic.theclinics.com

---

**Box 1**
**Hyperhidrosis disease severity scale**

*"How would you rate the severity of your hyperhidrosis?"*

1. My sweating is never noticeable and never interferes with my daily activities.
2. My sweating is tolerable but sometimes interferes with my daily activities.
3. My sweating is barely tolerable and frequently interferes with my daily activities.
4. My sweating is intolerable and always interferes with my daily activities.

---

This review focuses on therapies that have been approved or cleared by the US Food and Drug Administration (FDA) and potential treatments that are undergoing promising clinical investigation.

## CHEMODENERVATION

Although several botulinum toxins are commercially available with published data on treating hyperhidrosis, only onabotulinumtoxin A (onabotA), (BOTOX; Allergan Inc, Irvine, California), was FDA approved in 2004 for the treatment of severe primary axillary hyperhidrosis in adults. Numerous studies show the efficacy and safety of onabotA to treat axillary hyperhidrosis. One multicenter, randomized, controlled, double-blind study, compared effects of onabotA with placebo in 320 subjects 18 and older. This study found that greater than 90% of participants experienced at least a 50% reduction in axillary sweating 4 weeks after treatment.[4] The safety profile of onabotA was similar to that in the placebo group.

Another study evaluated the efficacy and safety of onabotA in adolescents ages 12 to 17 years with severe primary axillary hyperhidrosis. Up to 72% of patients experienced at least a 2-grade improvement in the HDSS score at 4 and 8 weeks after each of the first 2 treatments.[5] The median duration of effect ranged from 134 to 152 days. Less than 6% of patients experienced treatment-related adverse effects.[5] Overall, this study found that the efficacy and safety of onabotA can also be extended to adolescents.

Botulinum toxins can be used off label to treat hyperhidrosis in other body regions, including but not limited to the face/scalp, inguinal region, or palms/soles.[6,7] Each anatomic location presents unique challenges, but in the palms, the injections tend to cause more pain and can be associated with risk of muscle weakness when injecting over the thenar eminence.[7]

Possible new topical formulations of botulinum toxin are under investigation by at least 2 different companies, Revance Therapeutics (Newark, California) and Transdermal Corp (Birmingham, Michigan).

Glogau's randomized, blinded, vehicle-controlled study of 12 patients using 200 U of onabotA in a proprietary vehicle delivery system developed by Revance Therapeutics found a statistically significant 65% reduction in sweating reported at 4 weeks compared with 25.3% in the vehicle-treated axilla.[8] No systemic adverse events were reported, and very few local adverse events were observed, none of which were considered related to the treatment.

A second company, Transdermal Corporation, is developing a topical agent based on ionic nano-particle technology.[9] This agent consists of micelles that entrap the active ingredient with no changes in its chemical composition; this creates particles that are smaller than skin pores. Data from clinical trials are scarce, and more information is needed to evaluate its efficacy in hyperhidrosis.

## TAP WATER IONTOPHORESIS THERAPY

Tap water iontophoresis is a first line option to treat palmoplantar hyperhidrosis, a lifelong, socially embarrassing, and occupationally disabling condition. Iontophoresis uses the passage of a direct electrical current onto the skin and can serve as an effective treatment option. Side effects are typically minor and related to higher amperage. Skin erythema, minor pain or paresthesias in the treated areas, and minor burns can occur.[10] For patients who have any breaks in the skin, it is recommended to apply petroleum jelly to those areas to reduce irritation and the passage of current through the open skin. The underlying mechanism of iontophoresis is not fully understood. One hypothesis is that iontophoresis may induce a hyperkeratotic plug in the eccrine duct and obstruct sweat flow and secretion.[11] Another proposed mechanism includes impairment of the electrochemical gradient of sweat secretion.

Tap water iontophoresis should be performed every 48 to 72 hours. Successful reduction in sweating usually requires the application of 15 to 20 mA.[12] Each treatment takes approximately 30 to 40 minutes to perform (15–20 minutes for the palms and 15–20 minutes for the soles). We generally suggest treating one hand and one foot together, so one free hand is available to control the unit (**Fig. 1**). Once therapeutic effect is achieved, treatments can be performed once weekly for maintenance. A controlled trial of 112

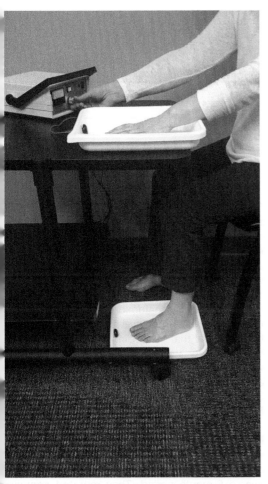

**Fig. 1.** A patient using the R.A. Fischer device to treat one hand and one foot simultaneously while using the second hand to control the panel.

patients with palmar hyperhidrosis showed that sweating was reduced by 81.2% from baseline with use of iontophoresis therapy.[10]

There are 3 iontophoresis devices that are registered with and cleared by the FDA; the R.A. Fischer and the Hidrex USA devices require a prescription, whereas the Drionic device is available without a prescription. The R.A. Fischer and the Hidrex USA both produce 2 different devices, and the comparison of pricing and similarities and differences between each device can be found on the manufacturer web sites.

## MICROWAVE ENERGY THERMOLYSIS

Cleared by the FDA in February of 2011 for primary axillary hyperhidrosis, miraDry (Miramar Labs, Inc, Sunnyvale, California), is the only nonsurgical device that can provide potentially permanent reduction in sweating. Microwave energy is delivered into the skin, generating heat to destroy eccrine sweat glands, but it is not selective and can affect the apocrine glands as well. Eccrine sweat glands do not regenerate, and their destruction could permanently abort sweating in the treated area. Microwave energy is readily absorbed by water molecules, and as a result, can easily target tissues with high water content, such as the sweat glands.[13] The energy absorption of miraDry is lowest in the epidermis and maximal at the derma/fat interface, independent of skin thickness.[14] Additionally, the device provides a cooling system that protects the superficial epidermis by inhibiting upward thermal conduction from the target energy absorption region.[14]

The miraDry device consists of a console, a handpiece, and a single-use biotip applicator, which uses a vacuum system to stabilize the skin during energy delivery. There are 5 energy settings; the power remains constant across all energy settings, and time is used to adjust the amount of energy delivered.[15] Axillary hair must be removed before treatment, and generally a nonsteroidal anti-inflammatory drug, such as ibuprofen, is administered 1 to 2 hours before the procedure, to minimize posttreatment swelling and discomfort.

A starch-iodine test can be performed to identify the precise location of sweating (**Fig. 2**). If no sweating is present at the time of the test, the entire hair-bearing area in the axillary vault should be treated. A supplied grid is used to measure the appropriate treatment area, and a temporary template is applied to the axilla corresponding to the size of the measurement obtained by the grid (**Fig. 3**).

Local anesthesia is necessary, and the original protocol called for injection of lidocaine 1% and epinephrine 1:100,000 up to a maximum dose of 7 mg/kg, approximately 1 cm apart along the marked areas on the temporary template. Coleman[16] developed an alternative method using high volumes of diluted lidocaine solution (high-volume anesthesia [HVA]), analogous to tumescent lidocaine anesthesia (**Table 1**).[16] This method allows for fewer needle sticks, good pain control, and maintained efficacy of the microwave thermolysis.

If using standard local lidocaine anesthesia, 2 treatment sessions are generally performed approximately 3 months apart. Lower energy levels are used at the superior axillary pole to reduce the risk of nerve injury. With the use of HVA, the authors treat at energy level of 5, decreasing or even eliminating the need for a second treatment. Although the risk of nerve injury is low, HVA may create a protective buffer space,

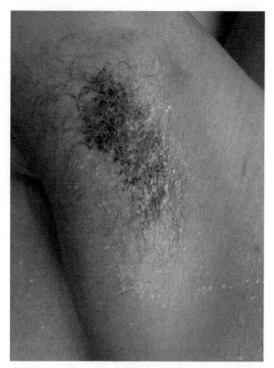

**Fig. 2.** A positive starch iodine test result in a patient with primary axillary hyperhidrosis. The starch iodine test can be performed without shaving axillary hair, but clean shaven axilla may be required for some procedures, such as miraDry thermolysis.

| Table 1 | |
|---|---|
| **Components of HVA for use before treatment with miraDry** | |
| **Ingredient** | **Amount** |
| 0.9% NaCl solution | 500 mL |
| 1% Lidocaine | 50 mL |
| 1:1000 epinephrine | 0.5 mL |
| 8.4% Bicarbonate | 5 mL |
| 10 mg/mL Triamcinolone | 0.5 mL |

shifting the neurovascular structures deeper into the axilla.

Common and temporary side effects of this procedure include edema, erythema, ecchymosis, and axillary tenderness/pain, which can last for several days.[17] Additionally, altered sensation in the axilla and occasionally extending down the arm can occur and last for approximately 5 weeks.[17] Patchy alopecia in the treated area is the only long-lasting and likely permanent side effect that has been reported. Less common side effects include blistering at the treatment site, skin irritation, and palpable axillary bumps, all of which resolve with time. More rarely, nerve injury has been reported owing to the median and ulnar nerves' superficial anatomic location after branching off the brachial plexus at the axillary level.[15] It is hypothesized that thinner individuals may be at a higher risk for temporary neuropathy compared with those with more subcutaneous fat in the axilla.[15] However, as mentioned earlier, the risk of nerve injuries may potentially be reduced with HVA.

Overall, miraDry is proving to be an effective and long-lasting solution in decreasing underarm sweating. Hong and Lupin[18] conducted a study on 31 patients who had 1 to 3 procedure sessions over a 6-month period. They reported approximately 90% overall efficacy persisting after 12 months.[18] At 12 months, 90.3% of patients had HDSS scores of 1 or 2, 90.3% had at least a 50% reduction in axillary sweat from baseline, and 85.2% had a reduction of at least 5 points on the Dermatology Life Quality Index questionnaire.[18] Two years after treatment, they found that 100% of subjects reported reduction in their HDSS scores to 1 or 2, although only 19 of 31 patients completed the final follow-up survey.[19]

## EXTERNALLY APPLIED ULTRASOUND THERAPY

A novel device using high-intensity microfocused ultrasonography plus visualization (MFU-V) to produce thermal coagulation points within the dermis at a specified depth has been undergoing investigation for the treatment of primary focal hyperhidrosis.[20] The Ulthera system (Ulthera Incorporated, Mesa, Arizona) has already been cleared by the FDA for skin tightening and lifting procedures.[21] For the treatment of axillary hyperhidrosis, the ultrasound energy is delivered to a

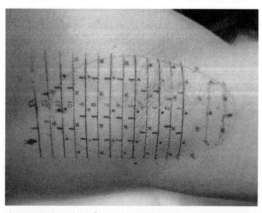

**Fig. 3.** Example of an appropriately sized miraDry template transferred onto the axilla before treatment.

specific depth in the skin up to 4.5 mm.[22] The visualization component of the device allows the user to avoid critical structures, such as large blood vessels and nerves during the treatment.

In 2014, Nestor and Park[20] reported results of 2 randomized, double-blind, sham-controlled pilot studies to assess the safety and long-term efficacy of MFU-V in treating axillary hyperhidrosis.[20] The first study consisted of 2 groups; 11 patients were assigned to group A and 3 patients to group B. Group A received 2 MFU-V treatments on one randomly chosen axilla and 2 sham treatments on the other axilla 30 days apart. Group B received 2 MFU-V treatments on both axillae 30 days apart. This group was also used to study the effect of subcutaneous lidocaine on level of discomfort and treatment efficacy. More than 50% of patients achieved a positive treatment response, and there was no difference in the reduction of sweat production among axillae that received subcutaneous lidocaine with or without epinephrine versus no pretreatment anesthesia.[20]

In the second study, 20 patients were randomly assigned to either bilateral MFU-V (N = 12) or sham treatment (N = 8). Baseline sweat production decreased by ≥50% in the MFU-V group but not in the sham group.[20]

Reported adverse effects were mild, and there were no serious or unexpected adverse events recorded. The most common side effects included tenderness or soreness in the axilla, reported by 86% of patients, and on average lasted approximately 11 days.[20]

Larger clinical studies are needed to formulate a firm conclusion on the efficacy and safety of this treatment, although the preliminary results seem promising.

## LASER THERAPY

There has been increasing interest in the use of laser therapy to treat axillary hyperhidrosis. This mode of treatment is again targeted at destroying sweat glands and theoretically can provide permanent sweat reduction.

### 1064-nm, 1320-nm, and 1440-nm Neodymium-doped Yttrium Aluminium Garnet Laser

Between May 2008 and November 2010, a retrospective study was conducted at a single center in Croatia, which included 32 patients who received treatment with a subdermal 1064-nm neodymium-doped yttrium aluminium garnet (Nd:YAG) laser for axillary hyperhidrosis.[23] Laser energy of approximately 200 J/cm$^2$ was delivered to sweat-producing areas, and the sweat glands

were removed with a suction probe (modified Blugerman-Schavelzon model).[23] Most patients (84%) reported reduction in their sweating as greater than 50%, and 22% of this group said their improvement was greater than 75%.[23] The reduction in sweating was stable over a 24-month period. Reported adverse effects were mild and transient, consisting of edema, pain, pulling sensation, and few cases of hematomas. There was also one case of partial skin erosion, which was medically treated and fully resolved 4 weeks after treatment.[23] Although this study was small and retrospective, it does illustrate promising efficacy in using a 1064-nm Nd:YAG laser subdermally to treat axillary hyperhidrosis.

A reported case of a 39-year-old African-American woman with refractory axillary hyperhidrosis, previously treated with topical aluminum chloride, botulinum toxin A, and thoracic sympathectomy without satisfactory resolution of symptoms was treated with a subdermal 1320-nm Nd:YAG laser at 30 Hz and 10 W. A total of 8810 J were delivered to both axillae with no adverse effects reported, and complete resolution of symptoms was maintained at 18 months.[24] The investigator hypothesized that the 1320-nm wavelength may be more effective than 1064-nm wavelength because of its ability to deliver more dermal energy absorption to where the eccrine glands reside.[25]

A prospective, nonrandomized study of 15 patients with axillary hyperhidrosis assessed reduction in sweating based on HDSS after using a 1400-nm Nd:YAG laser. Of the 15 patients treated, 3 reported an HDSS score of greater than 2 and required a second treatment 6 months after the initial treatment.[26] HDSS score decreased by 2.2, 1.8, and 1.9 points at 3 months, 6 months, and 12 months, respectively.[26] Additionally, histologic evaluation showed eccrine gland necrosis after laser treatment. Adverse effects included numbness, pain, erythema, swelling, bruising, and itching and were experienced by greater than 73% of patients, lasting only 2 to 3 days.[26]

### 924-nm and 975-nm Diode Laser

Leclere and colleagues[27] conducted a randomized, prospective, controlled trial to evaluate the efficacy of subdermal delivery of a diode laser using wavelengths of 924 nm and 975 nm. These wavelengths have a high affinity for water and can easily penetrate the superficial dermis and subcutaneous tissue, respectively. The investigators randomly divided 100 patients into 4 groups with 25 patients in each group: laser therapy alone at 975 nm (group 1), laser alone at 924/975 nm simultaneously (group 2), curettage alone (group 3), and finally laser at 924/975 nm followed by curettage (group 4).[27] HDSS, starch iodine test, and Global Aesthetic Improvement Scale were used to assess treatment efficacy. The results showed that 924/975-nm wavelengths combined with curettage was the optimal treatment option for axillary hyperhidrosis. Using the diode laser at 924-nm alone produced the least effective results, which may be related to a more superficial penetration. Combining both wavelengths allowed for penetration into the superficial dermis and deeper tissue. Using this technique with curettage-suction produces additional damage to the area, optimizing the results. Epidermal burns were the most significant complication in 2 patients treated with the 975-nm laser; it took 6 weeks to heal and left a permanent scar.[27] Other complications were temporary, persisting less than a month.

### Long-pulsed 800-nm Diode Laser

Bechara and colleagues[28] used a long-pulsed 800-nm diode laser to evaluate the effect of standard hair removal protocol on sweat rate of 20 patients with axillary hyperhidrosis. In this half-side–controlled trial, 5 treatment cycles were performed at 4-week intervals, using an energy setting of 50 mJ/cm$^2$ and pulse duration of 30 ms (1.6 Hz). Sweating was reduced, as measured by gravimetric assessment, from 89 mg/min and 78 mg/min at baseline to 48 mg/min and 65 mg/min 4 weeks after the last treatment in the treated and control axillae, respectively.[28] Histologic examination of skin biopsy sections before and after the laser treatment found no change in the number or size of apocrine or eccrine glands, and no damage to the glands was found. The only adverse effect noted was temporary axillary skin depigmentation in a single patient. The results were not statistically significant, and a larger sample size is needed to identify a therapeutic effect.

## TOPICAL ANTICHOLINERGICS

Anticholinergic agents inhibit the acetylcholine-induced activation of eccrine sweat glands.[10] Oral anticholinergic drugs have been used off label to treat primary multifocal hyperhidrosis, and although they can be effective, systemic side effects frequently limit their use and can include dry mouth, dry eyes, difficulty in urination, constipation, blurred vision, drowsiness, and dizziness. Several studies found positive results with topical glycopyrrolate ranging in concentrations from 0.5% to 2%. The authors found 1% topical glycopyrrolate compounded cream to be particularly effective for craniofacial hyperhidrosis. It is not

commercially available in the United States, but can be compounded at specialty pharmacies. A split-face study of 25 patients with craniofacial sweating, in which placebo was applied to one-half of their forehead and 2% topical glycopyrrolate was applied to the other half, found that 96% of patients were satisfied with the effectiveness of this agent.[29] Only one patient in this study was not able to tolerate treatment because of headache. Another study evaluated topical application of 0.5% or 1% glycopyrrolate in 16 patients with Frey syndrome (gustatory hyperhidrosis) and found that it was an effective treatment and free of adverse effects.[30]

Dermira Inc (Menlo Park, California), a specialty biopharmaceutical company studying a proprietary topical anticholinergic product (DRM04), has completed 2, phase 2b clinical trials in approximately 300 patients with severe, primary axillary hyperhidrosis. The first phase 2b study, completed in August 2014, found dose-dependent and, at certain doses, statistically significant results.[31] Average reduction in sweat production from baseline to week 4 ranged from 67.7% to 79.8% in patients treated with DRM04 compared with 48.7% in patients who received the vehicle only.[31] Additionally, 40.9% to 50.0% of patients achieved at least a 2-grade improvement in HDSS score from baseline to week 4 compared with 27.3% in those who received vehicle only. The results of the second phase 2b study were consistent with results of their previous study, and a phase 3 clinical trial is currently underway.

Brickell Biotech Inc (Miami, Florida), a clinical-stage pharmaceutical company working on the development of topical agents for hyperhidrosis, also completed a multicenter, randomized, double blind, vehicle-controlled phase 2b study, designed to evaluate the safety, tolerability, and efficacy of 3 concentrations of BBI-4000 (sofpironium bromide) gel versus vehicle in 189 subjects with primary axillary hyperhidrosis.[32] Sofpironium bromide is rapidly metabolized into a less-active metabolite by the time it reaches the blood stream, thus, potentially allowing for effective doses to be used topically while limiting systemic side effects.[32] Results from the phase 2b study showed BBI-4000 met its primary endpoint with a statistically significant 2-grade improvement in HDSS in a dose-related fashion and was well tolerated at all 3 concentrations studied.[32] Phase 3 studies have not been performed at the time of this writing.

Oxybutynin, which is another competitive muscarinic receptor antagonist, has been used topically off label for patients with hyperhidrosis. A new topical formulation of oxybutynin 3% topical gel was developed to increase tolerability of treatment of urinary incontinence compared with other transdermal formulations.[33] Adverse effects of topical oxybutynin gel are similar to those of topical glycopyrrolate and include skin irritation, dry mouth, constipation, headache, nasopharyngitis, and dizziness. There are no studies, however, that evaluated efficacy and safety of topical oxybutynin gel for focal hyperhidrosis, despite its off-label use in clinical practice.

## SUMMARY

A variety of treatment options are available for primary focal hyperhidrosis, and some can be combined for maximum effective results. Most therapies that have recently been FDA approved or cleared, such as miraDry, were only studied in axillary hyperhidrosis and cannot be used on other body areas. Topical anticholinergics, however, are being used off label on different body regions to treat hyperhidrosis and have shown promising results in smaller studies in treating craniofacial hyperhidrosis. There are also current clinical trials studying topical anticholinergic drugs in various concentrations and vehicles for treatment of axillary hyperhidrosis and soon might become another FDA-approved therapy option for patients who are not ready to pursue more invasive therapies. Despite the availability of these therapies, there is still a large need for new treatment options and studies on various body regions.

## REFERENCES

1. Glaser DA. A demographical analysis of hyperhidrosis. J Am Acad Dermatol 2007;56(2 Supp 2):AB46.
2. Basra M, Fenech R, Gatt R, et al. The dermatology life quality index 1994–2007: a comprehensive review of validation data and clinical results. Br J Dermatol 2008;159(5):997–1035.
3. Solish N, Bertucci V, Dansereau A. A comprehensive approach to the recognition, diagnosis, and severity-based treatment of focal hyperhidrosis: recommendations of the canadian hyperhidrosis advisory committee. Dermatol Surg 2007;33(8):908–23.
4. Naumann M, Lowe NJ. Botulinum Toxin Type A in treatment of bilateral primary axillary hyperhidrosis: randomised, parallel group, double blind, placebo controlled trial. BMJ 2001;323(7313):596–9.
5. Glaser DA, Pariser DM, Hebert AA, et al. A prospective, nonrandomized, open-label study of the efficacy and safety of onabotulinumtoxina in adolescents with primary axillary hyperhidrosis. Pediatr Dermatol 2015;32(5):609–17.
6. Komericki P, Ardjomand A. Hyperhidrosis of face and scalp: repeated successful treatment with botulinum toxin type A. Indian J Dermatol Venereol Leprol 2012;78(2):201–2.
7. Glaser DA, Hebert AA, Pariser DM, et al. Palmar and plantar hyperhidrosis: best practice recommendations and special considerations. Cutis 2007;79(5 Suppl):18–28.
8. Glogau R. Topically applied botulinum toxin type a for the treatment of primary axillary hyperhidrosis: results of a randomized, blinded, vehicle-controlled study. Dermatol Surg 2007;33:S76–80.
9. Available at: http://www.transdermalcorp.com/technology. Accessed February 16, 2016.
10. Karakoc Y, Aydemir EH, Kalkan MT, et al. Safe control of palmoplantar hyperhidrosis with direct current. Int J Dermatol 2002;41:602–5.
11. Hill AC, Baker GF, Jansen GT. Mechanism of action of iontophoresis in the treatment of palmar hyperhidrosis. Cutis 1981;28:69–70, 72.
12. Thomas I, Brown J, Vafaie J, et al. Palmoplantar hyperhidrosis: a therapeutic challenge. Am Fam Physician 2004;69(5):1117–21.
13. Glaser DA, Galperin TA. Local procedural approaches for axillary hyperhidrosis. Dermatol Clin 2014;32(4):533–40.
14. Johnson JE, O'Shaughnessy KF, Kim S. Microwave thermolysis of sweat glands. Lasers Surg Med 2012;44(1):20–5.
15. Suh DH, Lee SJ, Kim K, et al. Transient median and ulnar neuropathy associated with a microwave device for treating axillary hyperhidrosis. Dermatol Surg 2014;40(4):482–5.
16. Coleman WP III, Coleman WP IV. An alternative method of pain management for microwave treatment of primary axillary hyperhidrosis. Presented as an abstract and poster at 2014 ASDS Annual Meeting in San Diego, California, November 6-9, 2014.
17. Jacob C. Treatment of hyperhidrosis with microwave technology. Semin Cutan Med Surg 2013; 32(1):2–8.
18. Hong HC, Lupin M, O'Shaughnessy KF. Clinical evaluation of microwave device for treating axillary hyperhidrosis. Dermatol Surg 2012;38:728–35.
19. Lupin M, Hong HC, O'Shaughnessy KF. Long-term efficacy and quality of life assessment for treatment of axillary hyperhidrosis with a microwave device. Dermatol Surg 2014;40(7):805–7.
20. Nestor MS, Park H. Safety and efficacy of microfocused ultrasound plus visualization for the treatment of axillary hyperhidrosis. J Clin Aesthet Dermatol 2014;7(4):14–21.
21. Brobst RW, Ferguson M, Perkins SW. Ulthera: initial and Six Month Results. Facial Plast Surg Clin North Am 2012;20(2):163–76.
22. Laubach HJ, Makin IR, Barthe PG. Intense focused ultrasound: evaluation of a new treatment modality for precise microcoagulation within the skin. Dermatol Surg 2008;34:727–34.

23. Maletic D, Maletic A, Vizintin Z. Laser assisted reduction of axillary hyperhidrosis (LARAH) – evaluation of success up to 24 months after the treatment. J LAHA 2011;1:37–42.

24. Kotlus BS. Treatment of refractory axillary hyperhidrosis with a 1320-nm Nd:YAG laser. J Cosmet Laser Ther 2011;13(4):193–5.

25. Reszko AE, Magro CM, Diktaban T, et al. Histological comparison of 1064 nm Nd:YAG and 1320 nm Nd:YAG laser lipolysis using an ex vivo model. J Drugs Dermatol 2009;8:377–82.

26. Caplin D, Austin J. Clinical evaluation and quantitative analysis of axillary hyperhidrosis treated with a unique targeted laser energy delivery method with 1-year follow up. J Drugs Dermatol 2014;13(4):449–56.

27. Leclere FM, Moraga JM, Alcolea JM, et al. Efficacy and safety of laser therapy on axillary hyperhidrosis after one year follow-up: a randomized blinded controlled trial. Lasers Surg Med 2015;47:173–9.

28. Bechara FG, Georgas D, Sand M, et al. Effects of a Long-pulsed 800-nm diode laser on axillary hyperhidrosis: a randomized controlled half-side comparison study. Dermatol Surg 2012;38(5):736–40.

29. Kim WO, Kil HK, Yoon KB, et al. Topical glycopyrrolate for patients with facial hyperhidrosis. Br J Dermatol 2008;158:1094–7.

30. Hays LL. The frey syndrome: a review and double blind evaluation of the topical use of a new anticholinergic agent. Laryngoscope 1978;88:1796–824.

31. Dermira Announces Positive Phase 2b Results for DRM04 in Patients with Hyperhidrosis. Available at: http://dermira.com/dermira-announces-positive-phase-2b-results-for-drm04-in-patients-with-hyperhidrosis/. Accessed February 16, 2016.

32. Brickell Biotech Achieves Statistically Significant and Clinically Meaningful Phase 2b Results for BBI-4000 (Sofpironium Bromide) in Patients with Hyperhidrosis. Available at: http://brickellbiotech.businesscatalyst.com/12172015_BrickellBiotech.html. Accessed February 16, 2016.

33. Goldfischer ER, Sand PK, Thomas H, et al. Efficacy and safety of oxybutynin topical gel 3% in patients with urgency and/or mixed urinary incontinence: a randomized, double-blind, placebo-controlled study. Neurourol Urodyn 2013;34(1):37–43.

# Selecting the Right Patient for Surgical Treatment of Hyperhidrosis

Alan Edmond Parsons Cameron, MA, MCh, FRCS*

## KEYWORDS

- Sympathectomy • Hyperhidrosis • Patient selection

## KEY POINTS

- Endoscopic thoracic sympathectomy (ETS) is a good option for palmar sweating.
- It is not the first choice for axillary sweating and other operations may be preferred.
- ETS can be used for craniofacial sweating but only after very careful consideration.

## INTRODUCTION

The earliest sympathectomy was probably performed by Alexander in 1889 to treat epilepsy.[1] Surgery was tried for other indications, but the first successful sympathectomy for hyperhidrosis was reported by Kotzareff[2] in 1920; he cured a patient with severe unilateral cranial sweating and, since then, excessive sweating has been the most common indication for surgery.

In his 1850 novel, *David Copperfield*, Charles Dickens gave a splendid description of the ideal candidate for treatment.[3] Copperfield shakes the hand of the villainous Uriah Heep and then says "what a clammy hand his was. I rubbed mine afterward to warm it and to rub his off." Later he sees Heep's "lank forefinger leaving snail-like tracks upon the page." So that individual would definitely have been helped by surgery! These days, however, with a wider range of treatments and a wider spectrum of cases, selecting the right patient is more problematic.

Perhaps the easiest way to approach the subject is to consider the anatomic sites of sweating.

## PALMAR HYPERHIDROSIS
### Overview

Hand sweating remains the best indication for surgery and the only effective surgery is some attack on the sympathetic chain. Although originally this was done by open surgery,[4] it is now always by endoscopic thoracic sympathectomy (ETS). (See discussion of various surgical approaches to ETS, in this issue.) There is a variety of techniques using different instruments (eg, diathermy, harmonic scalpel, scissors, clipping, robotics) or by different anatomic approaches (eg, resection, ablation, ganglionectomy, ramicotomy). However, at the end of the day, the results seem broadly similar. What seems to matter is that the chain is damaged by some means. Of more relevance perhaps is the level at which the chain is attacked. (See discussion of growing consensus that in palmar sweating the highest level at the second rib is best avoided, in this issue.)

### Clinical Assessment

The ideal patient has an established history of severe palmar sweating interfering with work or social interaction.

Disclosure Statement: None.
Department of Surgery, Ipswich Hospital, Heath Road, Ipswich IP4 5PD, United Kingdom
* 4 Parkside Avenue, Ipswich IP4 2UL, United Kingdom.
E-mail address: alan.cameron@talktalk.net

Thorac Surg Clin 26 (2016) 403–406
http://dx.doi.org/10.1016/j.thorsurg.2016.06.004
1547-4127/16/© 2016 Elsevier Inc. All rights reserved.

thoracic.theclinics.com

The history of primary hyperhidrosis is characteristic; for example, sweating does not occur during sleep, which makes it easy to exclude any systemic causes.

Although there are questionnaires specifically designed for sweating,[5,6] most surgeons do not use these. Although there are quantitative methods of measuring sweat output, either gravimetric by weighing pads or electronic sudometers, these are cumbersome and only research tools so, again, they are not used in clinical practice.[7]

Sometimes perspiration can be observed dripping off the fingers, but the sweat output is very variable so usually the surgeon has to rely on the patient's description of the symptoms. The sweating is undoubtedly affected by emotion. Sweating causes anxiety that then increases the sweating and so a vicious cycle results. Many patients may have been prescribed antidepressants or anxiolytics, so it can be difficult for a surgeon to separate the emotional and physical aspects. This is particularly important when discussing surgery because some of these anxious patients are seeking perfection and may be very unhappy with even mild adverse side-effects.

There are options for the treatment of palmar sweating. Oral anticholinergics have been used since 1950[8] but efficacy is limited by side-effects.[9] Iontophoresis, introduced by Levit[10] in 1968 is effective but tedious. Botox has been used for control of sweating since 1994[11] but is painful on the hands.

So ETS can be regarded as treatment of last resort and it is vital to ensure that any prospective candidate for surgery has been fully informed of the risks and consequences of ETS.[12] Informed consent has always been part of a surgeon's duty of care to any patient, but in these litigious days it is now also essential for self-preservation.

### Contraindications

There are relatively few contraindications to surgery. Although pediatricians and dermatologists dislike the operation, ETS can be done in children once they are large enough to get the instrument easily through the ribs and there do not seem to be any long-term consequences.[13] Palmar hyperhidrosis usually starts in childhood and does not get better, so there is no reason for delay to see if the child grows out of it. There is a genetic element, so sometimes parents who have had ETS as an adult will bring their child for early treatment so that the misery of adolescence with sweaty hands, which they themselves endured, can be avoided in their offspring.[14]

### Preoperative Assessment

Clearly general fitness is important, but most cases are fit young adults. A history of tuberculosis or of pneumothorax may predict intraoperative difficulties due to adhesions but need not be a contraindication. The presence of an azygos lobe can cause confusion intraoperatively, but this is rarely picked up on a routine on a chest radiograph.[15] Equally, although apical lesions of old tuberculosis may be seen, the commoner simple adhesions are not, so a preoperative chest radiograph is rarely of any value. Similarly, other preoperative tests are usually unnecessary but may be dictated by local anesthetic protocols.

### Summary

Although physicians, and especially dermatologists, often write about secondary hyperhidrosis, in practice such cases are exceedingly rare. The history of primary palmar hyperhidrosis is so characteristic that other conditions do not need to be excluded except in the most unusual circumstances.

So the most important part of selecting the patient for treatment is the informed discussion about the likely outcome of ETS and, in this respect, the operation is no different from any other. However, the procedure has a bad reputation among dermatologists, in particular, and critics see it as a lifestyle choice, forgetting that palmar sweating is a miserable condition for the sufferer. Surgeons, however, must acknowledge that some of the opposition is justified because previous indications may have been too liberal. Therefore, a surgeon is more than usually obliged to spell out clearly what is to be expected.

## PALMAR AND AXILLARY SWEATING
### Overview

If there is a combination of hand and armpit sweating, the selection of a patient for ETS is the same as for sweating confined to the hands. (See discussion of modification of surgery to include a lower level of the chain, in this issue.)

## ISOLATED AXILLARY SWEATING
### Nonsurgical Treatment

The right approach to the patient with sweating confined to the armpit is much more controversial and surgery has much less of a role.

Before considering any form of surgery it is important that all conservative measures have been shown to be ineffective. Thus the patient should have tried strong antiperspirants,[16] possibly with addition of steroid ointments to control inflammation.

Botox is probably the treatment of choice for isolated armpit sweating,[17] but some patients are seeking a more permanent cure rather than the repeated injections.

The new MiraDRY (Miradry. Miramar Labs, Inc, Santa Clara, CA) device is a semisurgical instrument that causes heat destruction of the subdermal tissues containing the sweat glands while cooling the skin to prevent damage. It is effective[18] but currently expensive and not widely available.

## Local Axillary Surgery

If these measures have failed to control the symptoms, surgery does become possible but ETS is by no means the preferred option. Local surgery to the axilla can provide good control of the symptoms without any risk of systemic side-effects. Again there are various approaches. Simple wide excision of the affected area that has been mapped out by Minor's starch iodine test is a straightforward operation but has the complications of delayed healing and unsightly scarring. Less invasive techniques, such as subdermal curettage, are alternatives; however, the choice of such local surgery will depend not only on the patient's preference but also on the surgeon's experience.[19]

## Role of Endoscopic Thoracic Sympathectomy

The early experience from Vienna[20] found that the results are much less satisfactory than for hand sweating alone and this is still current thinking. So ETS may be offered in selected cases but only after warning the patient that the results are much less satisfactory than for hand sweating.

Psychological factors seem less important in axillary than in hand sweating, but beware the patient who presents with a complaint that the armpits smell bad. Eccrine sweat glands produce a watery odorless secretion. If the patient complains of a bad smell, there may be issues other than body image and surgery of any kind is best avoided.

## PLANTAR HYPERHIDROSIS
### Types

Foot sweating can be isolated, concomitant with hand sweating, or a manifestation of post-ETS compensatory sweating. Most patients with concomitant foot and hand symptoms will opt for treatment of the hands, at least initially, and can be managed as previously discussed.

## Treatment

(See discussion of treatment of plantar sweating, in this issue.)

## CRANIOFACIAL SWEATING
### Clinical Aspects

This is the most contentious area for surgical treatment and selection of cases is extremely difficult.

Gross facial sweating is much more distressing than hand sweating. Because it cannot be hidden, many sufferers avoid occupations involving face-to-face contact with the public. Social interaction can be a nightmare. Many patients become profoundly depressed and anxious, often resorting to alcohol or drugs. Many are sent for hypnotherapy or counseling because it is perceived to be a psychological affliction. Paradoxically, this may have the unfortunate effect of simply making the patient think that it is somehow their own fault.

### Sympathectomy

The face does not lend itself to conservative treatment, so ETS may seem an attractive solution.

The difficulty, however, is that as shown by the review of more than 3000 cases treated by the Swedish group.[21] The long-term results for treatment of facial hyperhidrosis are less rewarding than for palmar symptoms and the regret rate increased over time.[21] The reason for this is actually unclear. It is correct that the highest level of the intrathoracic chain must be interrupted to get control of the facial symptoms.[22] This is usually referred to as the T2 level. (See fuller discussion, in this issue.) It may be that there is something special about this level of the chain that leads to bad consequences after division. Alternatively, it may be that patients with facial symptoms are inherently at risk of serious sequelae for the same reason that they got the symptoms in the first place.

### Caution

It is, therefore, essential to be extremely cautious in offering ETS to these patients. They are very distressed by their symptoms and desperate for a cure. Some of the information available on the Internet leads them to think that ETS will solve their craniofacial sweating without risk of long-term adverse consequences and, thereby, dramatically improve all aspects of their lives. Many such enquirers will be deterred once the risk of consequences has been pointed out. A small proportion will still wish to proceed. These should be the most severely handicapped only because only those with the most severe preoperative symptoms will accept the postoperative changes.[23]

### SUMMARY

The art of obtaining a successful outcome from any type of surgical intervention is to have the correct procedure done on the correct patient by the correct surgeon. This is vital for the often criticized surgical management of hyperhidrosis and there is no substitute for eternal vigilance.

## REFERENCES

1. Alexander W. The treatment of epilepsy. Edinburgh (United Kingdom): Pentland; 1889. p. 228.
2. Kotzareff A. Resection partielle du tronc sympathetic cervical droit pour hyperhidrosie unilateral (regions faciale, cervicale, thoracic et brachial droites. Rev Med Suisse 1920;40:111–3.
3. Dickens C. The personal history, adventures, experience, and observation of David Copperfield the Younger of Blunderstone Rookery. London: Bradbury and Evans; 1850.
4. Adar R, Kurchin A, Zweig A, et al. Plamar hyperhidrosis and its surgical treatment; a report of 100 cases. Ann Surg 1977;186:34–41.
5. Panhofer P, Neumayer C, Zacherl J, et al. A survey and validation guide for health-related quality-of-life status in surgical treatment of hyperhidrosis. Eur Surg 2005;37(3):143–52.
6. Kamudoni P, Mueller B, Salek MS. The development and validation of a disease-specific quality of life measure in hyperhidrosis; the Hyperhidrosis Quality of life Index (HidroQOL©). Qual Life Res 2015;24(4): 1017–27.
7. Illigens BM, Gibbons CH. Sweat testing to evaluate autonomic function. Clin Auton Res 2015; 19(2):79–87.
8. Grimson KS, Lyons CK, Watkin WT, et al. Successful treatment of hyperhidrosis using banthine. J Am Med Assoc 1950;143(15):1331–2.
9. Bajaj V, Langtry JA. Use of oral glycopyrronium bromide in hyperhidrosis. Br J Dermatol 2007;157(1): 118–21.
10. Levit F. Simple device for treatment of hyperhidrosis by iontophoresis. Arch Dermatol 1968;98(5):505–7.
11. Bushara KO, Park DM. Botulinum toxin and sweating. J Neurol Neurosurg Psychiatry 1994;57(11): 1437–8.
12. Ojimba TA, Cameron AEP. Drawbacks of endoscopic thoracic sympathectomy. Br J Surg 2004; 91(3):264–9.
13. Kao MC, Lee WY, Yip KM, et al. Palmar hyperhidrosis in children: treatment with video endoscopy laser sympathectomy. J Pediatr Surg 1994;29:387–91.
14. Ro KM, Cantor RM, Lange KL, et al. Palmar hyperhidrosis: evidence of genetic transmission. J Vasc Surg 2002;35(2):382–6.
15. Nelson HP, Simon G. The accessory lobe of the azygos vein. Br Med J 1921;1(3652):9–11.
16. Shelley WB, Hurley HJ Jr. Studies on topical antiperspirant control of axillary hyperhidrosis. Acta Derm Venereol 1975;55(4):241–60.
17. Naumann M, Lowe NJ. Botulinum toxin type A in treatment of bilateral primary axillary hyperhidrosis; randomised, parallel group, double blind, placebo-controlled trial. BMJ 2001;323(7313):596–9.
18. Schick CH, Grallath T, Schick KS, et al. Radiofrequency thermotherapy for treating axillary hyperhidrosis. Dermatol Surg 2016;42(5):624–30.
19. Wollina U, Kostler E, Schonlebe J, et al. Tumescent suction curettage versus minimal skin resection with subcutaneous curettage of sweat glands in axillary hyperhidrosis. Dermatol Surg 2008;34:709–16.
20. Herbst F, Plas EG, Fugger R, et al. endoscopic thoracic sympathectomy for primary hyperhidrosis of the upper limbs; a critical analysis and long term results of 480 operations. Ann Surg 1994;1: 86–90.
21. Smidfelt K, Drott C. Late results of endoscopic thoracic sympathectomy for hyperhidrosis and facial blushing. Br J Surg 2011;98(12):1719–22.
22. Cerfolio RJ, de Campos JR, Bryant AS, et al. The Society of Thoracic Surgeons expert consensus for the surgical treatment of hyperhidrosis. Ann Thorac Surg 2011;91(5):1642–8.
23. De Campos JR, Kauffman P, Werebe EC, et al. Quality of life, before and after thoracic sympathectomy: report on 378 operated patients. Ann Thorac Surg 2003;76:886–91.

# Targeting the Sympathetic Chain for Primary Hyperhidrosis
## An Evidence-Based Review

Joel M. Sternbach, MD, MBA[a], Malcolm M. DeCamp, MD[b],*

**KEYWORDS**

- Hyperhidrosis • ETS • Endoscopic thoracic sympathectomy • Sympathicotomy • Sympathotomy
- Sympathetic surgery • Compensatory sweating

**KEY POINTS**

- Long-term resolution of palmar hyperhidrosis can be expected in greater than 95% of appropriately selected patients undergoing endoscopic thoracic sympathicotomy (ETS).
- Axillary hyperhidrosis and craniofacial hyperhidrosis, separate disease entities, tend to have lower rates of treatment success than palmoplantar hyperhidrosis after ETS, resulting in patient satisfaction rates of 70% to 90% and 60% to 80%, respectively.
- Studies have consistently demonstrated a correlation between the extent of sympathetic interruption, number of levels targeted, and higher cephalic extent of interruption, and the degree of resolution of hyperhidrosis but also increased rates and severity of compensatory hyperhidrosis (CH).
- The operative approach should be individualized to address the preference of each patient regarding degree of palmar dryness desired versus willingness to accept the risk of CH.

## INTRODUCTION

Since Lin reintroduced the technique of thoraco-scopic sympathectomy in 1990,[1] the modern era of sympathetic surgery for the treatment of focal primary hyperhidrosis has seen incremental prog-ress driven mainly by single-center, retrospective case series. The lack of a common vocabulary to describe the method of interrupting the sympa-thetic chain and anatomic basis used to identify the location of interruption limited the ability to compare outcomes. The Society of Thoracic Surgeons Hyperhidrosis Task Force and Interna-tional Society on Sympathetic Surgery released a consensus statement in 2011 establishing a com-mon language for describing operative technique,

providing recommendations for where to interrupt the sympathetic chain based on presenting symp-toms and recommending standardization of the documentation of preoperative and postoperative symptomatic evaluation.[2]

The aim of this article is to review nomenclature, anatomy, and relevant anatomic variations of the sympathetic chain and provide an overview of clinical and anatomic studies regarding technical aspects of the operation, including patient posi-tioning, instrument selection, and intraoperative monitoring. Additions to the literature regarding palmar hyperhidrosis, axillary hyperhidrosis, and craniofacial hyperhidrosis since the release of the consensus statement in 2011 are reviewed with evidence-based recommendations for location,

[a] Department of Surgery, Northwestern University Feinberg School of Medicine, 251 East Huron Street, Suite 3-150, Chicago, IL 60611, USA; [b] Division of Thoracic Surgery, Northwestern Memorial Hospital, Northwestern University Feinberg School of Medicine, 676 North Saint Clair Street, Suite 650, Chicago, IL 60611, USA
* Corresponding author.
*E-mail address:* mdecamp@nm.org

Thorac Surg Clin 26 (2016) 407–420
http://dx.doi.org/10.1016/j.thorsurg.2016.06.005
1547-4127/16/© 2016 Elsevier Inc. All rights reserved.

method, and extent of sympathetic chain interruption offered.

## NOMENCLATURE

The following definitions are used in this review, based on the consensus recommendation to adopt a system based on rib level for describing the targeted segment of the sympathetic chain[2]:

- ETS: interruption of the sympathetic chain
- Endoscopic sympathetic block (ESB) or clipping: interruption of the transmission of nerve impulses along the sympathetic chain without division, usually accomplished with the application of endoscopic clips at 1 or more levels.
- Sympathectomy or ganglionectomy: excision of a portion of the sympathetic chain containing 1 or more ganglia; for example, an R3-R5 sympathectomy describes division of the chain at the third (R3), fourth (R4), and fifth (R5) ribs with either excision or ablation of the intervening third thoracic (T3) and fourth thoracic (T4) ganglions.
- Sympathotomy: division of the sympathetic chain without ganglion removal
- Ramicotomy: selective division of the rami communicantes, leaving the associated level of the sympathetic trunk intact
- Ablation: obliteration of a segment of the sympathetic chain, typically targeting 1 or more of the thoracic ganglia and most commonly accomplished with electrocautery

In addition, the lack of consistent terminology regarding what constitutes CH has limited the ability to compare surgical outcomes and contributed to published rates of CH after ETS, ranging from 10%[3] to as high as 98%[4] or 100%.[5] Investigators have cited both seasonal variation (CH most severe during the first summer after ETS[6]) and geographic variation in ambient temperature (100% rate of CH in a Brazilian cohort[7]) as further complicating factors in comparing published rates of CH. The consensus statement recommends standardizing classification of postoperative compensatory sweating into 3 categories[2]:

- Mild CH: a small amount of sweating, triggered by ambient heat, psychological stress, or physical exercise. The sweat that forms does not flow, is tolerable, and does not cause embarrassment or the need to change clothes.
- Moderate CH: sweating related to the triggers, listed previously, and that coalesces into droplets that flow, although not necessitating a change of clothes. Therefore, the

sweating, although uncomfortable, does not embarrass the patient.
- Severe or intense CH: large amounts of sweating in response to minimal or without ambient heat, psychological stress, or physical exercise. The sweat droplets that form flow profusely, requiring a change of clothes 1 or more times a day.

## COMPENSATORY HYPERHIDROSIS

Two main theories have been suggested regarding the cause of new-onset sweating in other areas of the body after ETS (most commonly affecting the back, chest, thighs, abdomen, groins, and feet):

- Reflex theory: attributes CH to an imbalance of positive and negative feedback signals within a hypothalamic reflex arc, due to disruption of afferent fibers in the sympathetic trunk, most likely those passing through the second thoracic (T2) ganglion[3,6]
- Redistribution theory: suggests the pathophysiology of CH includes at least a partial role for thermoregulatory redistribution of sweating to maintain preoperative levels. Recent data from Heidemann and Licht[8] showing CH in 25% of patients undergoing local surgical treatment of axillary hyperhidrosis (skin excision or liposuction/curettage) support the redistribution theory, as do reports of the occurrence of CH after axillary botulinum toxin injections for the treatment of focal hyperhidrosis.[9]

Despite the lack of consensus regarding the cause of CH, current evidence suggests that

- The higher the level of interruption of the sympathetic chain, the worse the CH (and rates of patient regret)[7]
  ○ Studies have consistently shown that interruption at the level of the T2 ganglion (second rib [R2] sympathotomy or R2-R3 sympathectomy) results in a higher incidence and severity of CH than disruption at lower levels.[10–14]
- The more extensive the destruction/interruption of the sympathetic chain, both in terms of technique and number of levels,[15] the higher the incidence and severity of CH
  ○ CH has been reported as less common in patients undergoing 1-level or 2-level interruption of the sympathetic chain compared with those undergoing 3-level denervation during ETS.[16–19]
  ○ Bryant and Cerfolio[20] recently reported the outcomes for 173 patients undergoing R2 and R3 versus isolated R4 or R4 and R5

sympathotomy. At a median follow-up of 6.9 years, "clinically bothersome" CH was reported by 74% of patients undergoing R2 and R3 sympathotomy and only 26% of patients in the R4 and R5 group.

For patients who are apprehensive about the risk of CH, prior to undergoing ETS, Miller and Force[21] suggest temporary sympathetic block with bupivacaine injection and proceeding to surgery in those patients who achieve an acceptable balance between resolution of hyperhidrosis and degree of compensatory sweating.

## ANATOMY OF THE SYMPATHETIC CHAIN

The sympathetic chain carries preganglionic fibers from the spinal cord as well as ascending and descending postganglionic fibers as it courses posteriorly through the neck and chest in a paravertebral location before terminating at the level of the second lumbar vertebrae. Typically described as a white cord visible beneath the parietal pleura, the sympathetic chain runs over the neck of the ribs near the articulation between each rib head and the vertebral column (**Figs. 1–3**). Anatomic studies consistently describe the significant variability of the sympathetic chain, both between individuals as well as between the right and left sides of any given patient. Atkinson and colleagues[22] reported encountering multiple sympathetic trunks in 6 of 155 patients undergoing ETS (all left sided), with 3 patients having 2 trunks and 3 patients having 3 trunks.

Zhang and colleagues[23] conducted a study of 25 adult cadavers focusing on the anatomic relationships of the sympathetic chain and found similar anatomy of the chain in only 4 (16%) of the cadavers studied. The stellate ganglion,

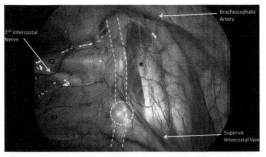

**Fig. 2.** Anatomy of the right apical sympathetic chain with anatomic relationships highlighted. (*) Fascia overlying the tendon of the longus coli muscle. (*Courtesy of* Dr Luiz Eduardo V. Leao, São Paulo, Brazil.)

formed by a fusion of the inferior cervical and first thoracic ganglia, was present in 80% of cases. The T2, T3, and T4 ganglia were most commonly located in the corresponding intercostal space (ICS) but with a notable downward shift of the ganglia relative to the ribs as the chain descended. This is reflected in the T2 ganglion located in the second ICS in 92% of the cadavers, whereas the T4 ganglion was located in the fourth ICS only 50% of the time, found along the upper border of the R5 in 36% of cases and positioned over the surface of the R5 in 10% of cases. Ramsaroop and colleageus[24] similarly reported finding the T2 ganglion below the inferior border of the R2 in 100% of cases.

Chiou and Liao[25] also evaluated the anatomy of T2 in 17 cadavers and described 2 anatomic relationships to assist with intraoperative localization of the sympathetic chain and T2:

- The superior intercostal artery was identified in 87.5% of cadavers, running parallel and lateral to the sympathetic chain at an average

**A**

**B**

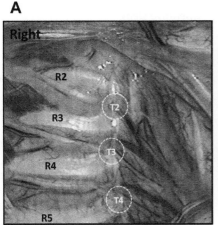

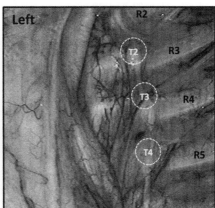

**Fig. 1.** Thoracoscopic view of the (*A*) right and (*B*) left sympathetic chains with rib number (R) and thoracic sympathetic ganglion number (T). (*Courtesy of* Dr Luiz Eduardo V. Leao, São Paulo, Brazil.)

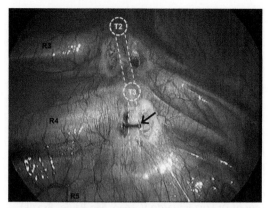

**Fig. 3.** Thoracoscopic image of the right sympathetic chain after application of a clip (*black arrow*) along the bottom edge of the R4. (*Courtesy of* Dr Luiz Eduardo V. Leao, São Paulo, Brazil.)

distance of 10 mm before terminating as the second intercostal artery

- The second intercostal nerve, part of the neurovascular bundle running along the lower border of the R2, can be traced directly to the T2 ganglion at its intersection with the sympathetic chain. In the right chest, the T2 ganglion is located lateral and superior to the azygos vein (see **Fig. 1**A). In the left chest, T2 can be found in the vicinity of the aortic arch, lateral to the hemiazygos vein (see **Fig. 1**B).

## Nerves of Kuntz

Referring to ascending rami between the second and first intercostal nerves that can provide an alternate pathway for postganglionic fibers to reach the brachial plexus, nerves of Kuntz (NK) are often implicated in cases of persistent or recurrent hyperhidrosis after ETS. A large discrepancy exists between the incidence of NK reported in clinical case series (10%[22]–38%[25]) and anatomic studies, describing the presence of NK 1 cm to 2 cm lateral to the sympathetic chain in 40% to 86% of cases.[23,24,26]

## ANATOMIC VARIATIONS AND SURGICAL PITFALLS
### Azygos Lobe

Baumgartner[27] described the rare occurrence of the sympathetic chain obscured by the presence of a congenital "azygos lobe," a weblike dome of tissue extending superiorly from the upper border of the azygous vein. In reviewing 1876 patients undergoing video-assisted thoracic sympathectomy for treatment of hyperhidrosis, Kauffman and colleagues[28] noted the presence of an azygos lobe

in 7 (0.37%) obscuring the T2 through T4 ganglia in all cases. They describe the pleural extension as similar to mesentery with a variable presence of intercostal vein branches. The investigators advocate the use of a double-lumen endotracheal tube (ETT) and the placement of an additional port as needed to facilitate visualization and dissection when an azygos lobe is encountered.

### Superior Intercostal Vein

Lee and colleagues[29] in a study of 23 cadavers noted the superior intercostal vein to cross the sympathetic chain in 22% of cases (see **Fig. 2**), with the most common location between the R4 and R5 (70%). In the right chest, the superior intercostal vein was noted to overly the T2 ganglion in 12% of cases, increasing the risk for bleeding during dissection in that area.[24]

### Fascia Overlying the Longus Colli Muscle

Particularly in thinner individuals, the band of white fascia overlying the longus colli muscle can be found tracking parallel to, and the same width as, the sympathetic chain in 10% of cases (see **Fig. 2**).[24,25] Located medial to the neck of the R2 the fascia was implicated by Singh and colleagues[30] as predisposing to technical failure in 0.5% of 786 sympathectomies for palmar hyperhidrosis.

## OPERATIVE TECHNIQUE

The steps of ETS are outlined in **Box 1** and include

- Patient positioning to optimize visualization of the sympathetic chain and minimize the risk of

---

**Box 1**
**Technical aspects of endoscopic thoracic sympathicotomy**

*Operative steps*

Semi-Fowler or supine positioning with chest elevated 45° to 70° and arms abducted less than 90°

Safe access to the chest cavity with single or multiple ports

Identification of sympathetic chain and any anatomic variants present

Dissection of the parietal pleura and interruption of the sympathetic chain

Lateral dissection 2–3 cm from the chain to divide any accessory nerves, if present

Reinflation of the lung under direct vision

Evacuation of residual capnothorax or pneumothorax

iatrogenic injury. Most commonly, ETS is performed in the semi-Fowler position or supine in steep reverse Trendelenburg position, with the chest elevated 45° to 70°. Arms are secured and abducted up to, but not beyond, 90° to prevent brachial plexus injury.[31] Rotation of a patient 20° to 30° away from the operative side can further assist in dropping the lung away from the superior sulcus.

- Safe access to the chest cavity with port placement designed to minimize trauma to the intercostal nerves and decrease the risk of postoperative intercostal neuralgia
- Identification of the sympathetic chain with attention to relevant landmarks and awareness of potential variations
- ETS or ESB, including lateral extension along the periosteum of the most cephalad level of interruption, to identify and divide any NK
- Consideration of the use of palmar temperature probes or Doppler blood-flow monitoring to detect successful reduction of sympathetic tone to the upper extremity
- Re-expansion of the lung under direct vision with a consistent method for evacuation/detection of pneumothorax or capnothorax

A variety of strategies for intubation have been described in case series, including the use of a double-lumen ETT allowing for single lung ventilation, single-lumen ETT with a bronchial blocker to isolate the operative side and single-lumen ETT with periods of intermittent apnea as needed to improve visualization during the case.[32,33] The use of low-pressure $CO_2$ insufflation can also assist in exposing the sympathetic chain. If used, most investigators recommend insufflation pressures less than 10 mm Hg to reduce the risk of hemodynamic compromise.[34]

Studies looking at specific aspects of the surgical approach to thoracoscopic sympathectomy have largely consisted of retrospective single-center series analyzing outcomes before and after a change in operative technique. Both Kuhajda and colleagues[34] and Kuijpers and colleagues[35] compared sequential lateral decubitus to the semi-Fowler positioning. Using the semi-Fowler positioning, which allowed both operative fields to be accessed without reprepping and draping the patients, resulted in a significantly shorter mean operative time (14–47 min vs 31–74 min) and avoided potential complications associated with repositioning an intubated patient.

Access to the chest is typically achieved with 2 ports placed in the axillae, between the second and sixth ICSs, with the superior or anterior port used for the thoracoscope and the other for the dissecting instrument. Uniportal techniques have also been described.[36]

Basic intraoperative monitoring for patients undergoing ETS should include noninvasive arterial blood pressure, electrocardiography, and pulse oximetry in all cases. Several investigators have studied the use of palmar temperature and/or Doppler blood flow monitors to detect a reduction in sympathetic tone.[15,22,37–41] Most investigators suggest a 1°C rise in temperature as indicative of successful denervation.

## METHOD OF INTERRUPTION
### Instrumentation

Several centers have reviewed differences in perioperative outcomes using electrocautery and ultrasonic/harmonic scalpel. Proposed advantages of ultrasonic instrument use include reduced smoke in the operative field and less thermal spread resulting in less-extensive damage to the sympathetic chain and decreased risk of injury to surrounding structures.[42,43] de Campos and colleagues[44] found no difference in pain scores at 1 week or 1 month in 929 patients undergoing ETS with electrocautery and 586 using a harmonic scalpel. A recent, smaller study[45] found the intensity of pain was higher with harmonic, in addition to acknowledging the increased cost. Weksler and colleagues[42] compared harmonic and cautery in 140 patients and found no evidence of difference in terms of complication rates, time to return to work, or clinical success rates between the two but commented on the decreased cost associated with the reusable hook electrocautery.

### Clipping

Lin and colleagues[46] initially described interruption of the sympathetic chain by clipping in 1998 in 326 patients with palmar hyperhidrosis. In a study comparing 80 male patients split evenly between resection, transection, ablation, and clipping, there were no differences in success rates but clipping had the shortest average operative time.[47] Coelho and colleagues[48] compared T3/T4 clipping versus sympathectomy in the treatment of axillary hyperhidrosis and found no significant differences in terms of treatment success, rates or severity of CH, or patient satisfaction. Panhofer and associates[49] more recently compared clipping at R4 and R5 with ETS using cautery at the same levels and found that clipping is less efficacious but results in decreased rates of CH, significantly so for plantar CH. Improvement in plantar hyperhidrosis was noted in 45.3% of ESB at R4 patients compared with 14.9% of ETS at R4 patients and "disturbing" CH in 9.9% (9 patients) in ETS group compared with 0.9% (1 patient) in ESB group.

The controversy surrounding reversibility of clipping is covered in detail elsewhere in this issue (See Conor F. Hynes and M. Blair Marshall's article, "Reversibility of Sympathectomy for Primary Hyperhidrosis," in this issue). As suggested in the Society of Thoracic Surgeons and International Society of Sympathetic Surgery consensus statement, without more definitive evidence in the interim to support reversibility, patients should be counseled that clipping is most likely permanent.[2]

### Sympathectomy Versus Sympathotomy

Aydemir and colleagues[50] compared T3 sympathectomy versus sympathicotomy and found the latter to have a significantly shorter operative time (50 min vs 36 min). Similar results were found by Mohebbi and colleagues[51] in comparing sympathectomy versus sympathicotomy at similar levels for hyperhidrosis occurring at a variety of sites and found a significantly longer operative time with sympathectomy (110.9 min vs 62.3 min, $P>.001$) as well as a significantly higher rate of CH in the sympathectomy group. Scognamillo and associates[52] also found sympathicotomy significantly faster than sympathectomy (15 min vs 28 min per side). During the study period (1993–2007), the investigators also noted that transition to smaller trocars (2 mm–5 mm) resulted in lower rates of intercostal neuralgia than 5 mm to 10 mm trocars (24% vs 46%).

### Ramicotomy

Hwang and colleagues[53] found selective R3/R4 ramicotomy to take significantly longer than R3 sympathotomy (51.6 min vs 19.8 min). The ramicotomy group had higher rates of persistent palmar hyperhidrosis and symptom recurrence and more severe lower extremity CH, resulting in significantly lower patient satisfaction (79.1% vs 91.3%). Ramicotomy was also noted by Lee and colleagues[54] and Kim and colleagues[55] to be associated with persistent or recurrent symptoms in as many as 30% to 32% of patients.

## LEVEL OF SYMPATHICOTOMY BASED ON SYMPTOMS

The past decade has seen a series of well-designed trials attempt to determine the optimal level and extent of sympathicotomy to balance resolution of hyperhidrosis with incidence and severity of compensatory sweating. The 2011 consensus guidelines, based on studies published through 2009, are outlined in **Table 1**, with recent

| Table 1 2011 Society of Thoracic Surgeons/ International Society of Sympathetic Surgery consensus recommendations | |
|---|---|
| **Location of Hyperhidrosis** | **Recommended Treatment Level** |
| Palmar | Either R3 or R4 |
| Axillary | Either R4 and R5 or R5 only |
| Palmar + axillary | R4 and R5 |
| Craniofacial | R3 or R2 and R3 |

additions to the literature based on primary location of presenting symptoms summarized in **Table 2** for palmar hyperhidrosis and **Table 3** for axillary hyperhidrosis.

One of the few areas where historical controversy seems to have been settled involves the exclusion of the lower third of the stellate ganglion in sympathectomy procedures for upper extremity hyperhidrosis, because no increase in efficacy could be demonstrated to justify the significant risk of Horner syndrome.[2,33]

### Palmar

For palmar hyperhidrosis, the recommended operation is sympathotomy or clipping of the sympathetic chain at the top of the R3. The recommendation is based on studies showing that R3 yields the driest hands; however, R4 interruption is also reasonable, usually resulting in mildly moist palms but decreased risk of CH.

Early studies presented conflicting data regarding the benefit of limiting the extent of sympathectomy, including those of Leseche and colleagues,[56] Moya and colleagues,[57] and Atkinson and colleagues.[22] More recently, 2 prospective randomized trials[7,33] have offered support for the concept of limited and lower sympathicotomy for palmar hyperhidrosis. Ishy and colleagues[7] randomized patients to R3-R4 or R4-R5 sympathectomy and achieved significant, objective decreases in palmar sweating in both groups to the level of normal controls at 1 week, 1 month, 6 months, and 1 year postoperatively. There was a trend toward slightly drier hands in the R3-R4 group at all time points but at 1-year that group reported a significantly higher rate of CH (100% vs 75% in the R4-R5 group, $P<.05$). The reported rate of severe CH for both groups (5% in R3-R4 and 7% in R4-R5) is lower than that reported in historical series in which higher-level interruption was performed.[58] The benefit of more caudal sympathicotomy was further supported by Baumgartner and

**Table 2**
Comparative studies for treatment of palmar hyperhidrosis

| Author, Year | Study Type | Patients (N) | Technique | Immediate Success Rate | Rate of Compensatory Hyperhidrosis | Follow-up (mo) | Recurrence Rate (%) |
|---|---|---|---|---|---|---|---|
| Ishy et al,[7] 2011 | Prospective randomized | 20 | R3-R4 Sympathectomy | 100% | 100% | 12 | 0 |
| | | 20 | R4-R5 Sympathectomy | 100% | 75% | 12 | 0 |
| Baumgartner et al,[33] 2011 | Prospective randomized | 61 | R2 Sympathotomy | 95.9% | 75.5% (2% severe) | 12 | 4.1 |
| | | 60 | R3 Sympathotomy | 95.8% | 58% (2% severe) | 12 | 4.2 |
| Hwang et al,[53] 2013 | Prospective, non-random (Patient choice) | 46 | R3 (bottom) Sympathotomy | 98% | 80.4% (disabling 8.7%; 10.9%) | 12 | 2.2 |
| | | 43 | R3 and R4 Ramicotomy | 84% | 95.3% (disabling 14%; 37.2%) | 12 | 16.3 |
| Kim et al,[59] 2010 | Retrospective | 56 | R3 Sympathotomy | 100% | 82.1% (7.1% moderate, 3.6% severe) | 22 | 3.2 |
| | | 63 | R4 Sympathotomy | 100% | 17.5% (3.2% moderate) | 22 | 1.8 |
| Abd Ellatif et al,[60] 2014 | Retrospective | 129 | R3 Sympathotomy | 100% (74.4% completely dry, 8.5% overly dry) | 74.4% (10% severe) | 19 | 0.8 |
| | | 145 | R4 Sympathotomy | 100% (33.2% completely dry, 0.7% overly dry) | 28.3% (0.7% severe)[a] P<.001 | 19 | 1.4 |
| Aoki et al,[32] 2014 | Retrospective | 25 | R2 or R3 Sympathotomy | 100% | 100% (less severe) | 20.3 | Not reported |
| | | 27 | R2 and R3 Sympathotomy | 100%[a] | 100% | 55.3 | Not reported |

[a] Lower average palmar sweat score, 0.8 versus 3.2, P<.01.

**Table 3**
Comparative studies for treatment of axillary hyperhidrosis

| Author, Year | Study Type | Patients (N) | Technique | Immediate Success Rate (%) | Rate of Compensatory Hyperhidrosis | Follow-up (mo) | Recurrence Rate (%) |
|---|---|---|---|---|---|---|---|
| Munia et al,[61] 2008 | Prospective randomized | 31 | R3-R5 sympathectomy | 100 | 100% | 12 | 0 |
| | | 33 | R4-R5 sympathectomy | 100 | 42% | 12 | 0 |
| Guimarães et al,[62] 2013 | Prospective randomized | 30 | R3, R4 and R5 clipping | 100 | 76.70% | 12 | 3.3 |
| | | 30 | R3 and R4 clipping | 100 | 83% | 12 | 0 |
| | | 30 | R4 and R5 clipping | 100 | 80% | 12 | 13.3 |
| Yuncu et al,[63] 2013 | Prospective randomized | 17 | R3 and R4 sympathotomy | 100 | 100% (35% grade 3, 47% grade 4) | 12 | 0 |
| | | 43 | R3 sympathotomy | 100 | 79% (23% grade 3, 35% grade 4) | 12 | 0 |
| Coelho et al,[48] 2009 | Retrospective | 42 | R3-R5 clipping | 83 | 78.6% (9.5% severe) | 24 | 0 |
| | | 42 | R3-R5 sympathectomy (ablation) | 93 | 76.2% (9.5% severe) | 24 | 4.8 |
| Heidemann & Licht,[8] 2013 | Retrospective | 28 | R2 and R3 sympathicotomy | 32 | 82% | 26 | 4 |
| | | 17 | R2, R3 and R4 sympathicotomy | 41 | 88% | 26 | 0 |
| | | 10 | En bloc skin resection | 90 | 50% | 26 | 25 |
| | | 30 | Suction-curettage | 63 | 17% | 26 | 60 |

colleagues[33] randomized trial comparing single-level R2 versus R3 sympathotomy in 121 patients with classic palmar hyperhidrosis. Although symptomatic relief was achieved in all patients, the R2 group had a significantly higher rate of CH (75.5% vs 58%). Similarly, in Yazbek and associates'[5] earlier trial, randomizing patients to single-level R2 or R3 sympathectomy, 100% of patients noted some degree of CH, but the R3 group reported significantly less severe CS (14% vs 46%, P = .007). Aoki and colleagues[32] compared outcomes of single level R2 or R3 versus R2/R3 sympathotomy in 52 patients with palmar hyperhidrosis. Although 100% of patients in both groups reported some degree of CH, the investigators reported single-level sympathotomy to be associated with a significantly lower severity on a scale of 1 (least severe) to 5 (most severe) (3.0 vs 4.0 for R2/R3, P<.01).

Moving further down the chain, Kim and colleagues[59] found that although the immediate success rate was 100% for single-level sympathotomy at either R3 or R4, overly dry palms occurred in only the R3 group (5.4%). Postoperative gustatory sweating was infrequent (4.2%) but also occurred only in the R3 group. There were no cases of patients regretting surgery in either arm, compared with rates of 2% to 50% seen in prior studies of interventions higher on the chain.[58] Abd Ellatif and colleagues[60] reviewed outcomes for 274 patients undergoing R3 or R4 sympathotomy for palmar hyperhidrosis at a mean follow-up of 19 months. The 2 groups had similar low recurrence rates (0.8% vs 1.4%) but the complaint of overly dry hands was noted in 8.5% of patients in the R3 group and only 0.7% (1 patient) in the R4 group. Axillary sweating also improved in 87.6% versus 100% in groups R3 and R4, respectively. CH was observed in 74.4% of the R3 group versus 28.3% with R4 sympathotomy and was reported as severe in 10% and 1.4%, respectively.

Based on the recent additions to the literature of evidence from prospective, randomized trials, an isolated R4 sympathotomy seems to achieve high rates of symptomatic relief for patients with isolated palmar hyperhidrosis without causing overly dry hands and with lower rates and severity of CH.

## Axillary

Citing results from the prospective, randomized trial by Munia and colleagues,[61] and earlier work by Chou and associates,[3] the 2011 consensus guidelines recommended an R4 and R5 sympathicotomy for the treatment of combined palmar-axillary or palmar-axillary-plantar symptoms or isolated axillary hyperhidrosis. An R5 interruption alone was also suggested as a viable option for patients with only axillary hyperhidrosis.

Guimarães and associates[62] randomized a total of 90 patients equally between 3 methods of ESB, R3-R5 clipping, R3-R4 clipping and R3-R4 clipping with addition of ramicotomy at the R3 level. All 3 groups achieved immediate symptomatic relief in 100% of patients but at 2-year follow-up, the group receiving the least extensive interruption (R3/R4 clipping) was the only one without recurrences. Rates of CH between the 3 groups did not differ significantly and ranged from 77% to 83%, comparable to the rates reported by Coelho and colleagues[48] for multilevel interruptions. Yuncu and colleagues[63] also found a significantly higher incidence and severity of CH as measured by the HDSS in patients undergoing more extensive interruption. Although the immediate success rate for patients in all 3 randomized trials was 100%, the group randomized by Munia and colleagues[61] to R4-R5 sympathectomy reported the lowest rate of CH.

For isolated axillary hyperhidrosis, Heidemann and Licht[8] recently showed improved outcomes with local treatment using subcutaneous liposuction/curettage or local skin excision compared with 2-level or 3-level sympathicotomy.[8] Recurrence rates were significantly higher in the local treatment group, particularly in the suction/curettage group (although the recurrent symptoms were predominantly mild with no patients requesting reoperation). The investigators found 25% of patients reported CH after local treatment, although the rates of CH for both R2 and R3 (82%) and R2-R4 (88%) ETS were significantly higher.

For combined palmar and axillary hyperhidrosis, either an isolated R4 or R4 and R5 sympathotomy seems to offer the optimal ratio of symptom resolution to compensatory sweating, while the work by Heidemann and Licht[8] provide compelling evidence that isolated axillary hyperhidrosis may be more effectively managed with local treatment modalities.

## Craniofacial

The 2011 consensus recommendations, based on a more limited set of available studies, suggest an R3 interruption or an R2 and R3 interruption for the treatment of primary craniofacial hyperhidrosis, acknowledging that the latter may lead to a higher incidence of CH, and increased risk of Horner syndrome, especially on the left side.[2]

Bell and colleagues[64] included 27 patients with craniofacial hyperhidrosis in the report of their outcomes after applying a standardized R2-R4 sympathotomy technique, regardless of presenting symptoms. Despite symptom resolution in 93%, the overall patient satisfaction rate was only 52%, likely related to the significantly higher incidence of troublesome or severe CH (44.5%) in patients presenting with craniofacial hyperhidrosis versus those patients with primarily axillary (26%) or palmar (8%) hyperhidrosis. Nicholas and colleagues,[65] in a recent systematic review, found R2 or R2 and R3 sympathicotomy to have a high rate of treatment success (70%–100% at mean follow-up of 29 months) but rates of troublesome CH ranging from 8% to 95.4% of patients.

Despite the historical emphasis on exclusion of the T2 ganglion, studies reporting on interruptions at lower levels of the chain have demonstrated success in treating craniofacial hyperhidrosis. Chou and associates[3] included 33 patients undergoing R3 and R4 clipping for facial hyperhidrosis in their series evaluating the outcomes of ESB. This lower level resulted in a 91% satisfaction rate, with compensatory sweating reported by only 27.3% of patients. Neumayer and associates[66] reported on the outcomes of 30 patients with facial hyperhidrosis that underwent ESB with clips at R3 and R4. Complete symptomatic relief was achieved in 82.8% of patients and another 10.3% reported a nearly dry face postoperatively. CH was reported by 27.6% and although gustatory sweating was present in nearly 60% of cases, it did not seem to adversely affect quality of life or overall satisfaction with the procedure (80% + 10% partial satisfaction).

Based on the results of these historical studies and those presented previously, showing sympathectomy at more cephalad levels is associated with increased operative time and complication rates, the current procedure of choice for isolated craniofacial hyperhidrosis appears to be a limited R3 sympathotomy.

## MECHANISMS OF FAILURE

Primary technical failure (either unilateral or bilateral) has been documented after ablation,[67] sympathectomy,[30,68] and clipping.[69] Persistent or recurrent symptoms can typically be attributed to issues with either the adequacy or accuracy of the initial operation:

- Inadequate: incomplete interruption during sympathotomy,[40] as a result of performing ramicotomy or due to insufficient compression with clipping to interrupt signaling along the sympathetic chain

- Inaccurate: failure to identify and divide accessory NK or recognize anatomic variation leading to interruption at an incorrect location

Errors of either type emphasize the importance of a thorough knowledge of relevant anatomy as well as lateral dissection along the periosteum for 2 cm at the chosen level of sympathicotomy. Options to help decrease the risk of failure in cases of ambiguous anatomy include obtaining intraoperative chest radiograph to confirm rib levels, performing a sympathectomy with histologic confirmation or the use of temperature or blood-flow monitoring to detect decrease in sympathetic tone.[30,36]

## REINTERVENTION

Symptomatic recurrence rates in the literature differ based on presenting symptoms and have ranged from 0% to 13.7% with varying length of follow-up, operative techniques, and levels of interruption of the sympathetic chain.[33,40,67,70,71]

Hsu and colleagues[40] reported the first series of 20 patients undergoing reoperation in 1998. Symptoms had recurred 3 to 18 months after the primary operation, and resympathectomy was successful in 15/15 (100%) of palmar cases and 4/5 (80%) of axillary cases. Due to the frequent presence of pleural adhesions in patients undergoing resympathectomy, the investigators recommend the use of a double-lumen ETT to allow for selective lung ventilation.

Licht and associates[70] described their experience with resympathicotomy (re-ETS) in 48 (7%) of 669 patients over a 10-year period; 35 of 36 patients (96%) with primary failure had symptomatic improvement with re-ETS. During reoperation, the investigators performed midrib division of the sympathetic chain at R2 and R3 for palmar hyperhidrosis and R2-R4 for axillary hyperhidrosis. Patients reported an 80% rate of CH after their primary operation and 38% described worsening of CH after re-ETS, in particular those patients treated for primary failure. At the time of re-ETS, Licht and colleagues[70] recommend extending the incision of the parietal pleura a few centimeters laterally to identify and destroy any previously missed accessory NK.

In their randomized trial comparing R2 and R3 sympathotomy for palmar hyperhidrosis, Baumgartner and colleagues[33] noted early and "dramatic" failure in 3 (5%) of the 60 patients in the R3 group. Two of the 3 patients presented with recurrence of dripping sweat at the palms in the first few weeks after surgery and underwent reoperation at the R2 level, resulting in complete symptomatic relief at 12-month follow-up.

Freeman and colleagues[71] reported on their reoperative experience over a 6-year period in 40 patients (87.5% refractory and 12.5% recurrent); 25% of the patients had previously undergone percutaneous ablation, with all failures in that group attributed to inaccurate localization. The investigators used a single-lumen ETT with a bronchial blocker and low-pressure $CO_2$ insufflation to improve visualization and performed an R3 sympathectomy, regardless of the initial procedure. Two 5-mm ports were used, but the investigators advocate the use of a third port for retraction of the lung in cases where dense pleural adhesions are encountered (more common in elderly patients and reoperative cases). Patients undergoing re-ETS had a significantly higher rate of moderate to severe CH (53% vs 31%, $P = .01$). A higher incidence of pleural adhesions was likely responsible for an increased frequency of pleural drainage and associated increases in hospital length of stay in patients undergoing re-ETS. Lin and colleagues[67] similarly encountered pleural adhesions in 14/24 (58.3%) patients undergoing re-ETS. In a follow-up study reporting the outcome of 42 patients undergoing re-ETS, Lin[39] noted CH in 86% of patients after reintervention.

## SUMMARY

Recent additions to the extensive literature on ETS for palmar hyperhidrosis suggest that single-level, limited sympathotomy at the level of the R4 results in subtotal sympathetic denervation, providing satisfactory relief of sweating while minimizing the incidence and severity of CH. For the treatment of isolated axillary hyperhidrosis, local surgical treatments, especially en bloc skin resection, seem to offer a high rate of initial symptomatic relief with significantly lower rates of CH compared with traditional multilevel ETS, although recurrence rates of 25% to 60% suggest the need for longer-term studies. For those patients opting for ETS or ESB to treat axillary or palmar-axillary hyperhidrosis, limiting the extent of interruption to R4 or R4-R5 may result in improved patient satisfaction related to decreased incidence of severe CH.

Recent data support the theory by Lin and Telaranta[6] that the T2 ganglion is implicated in the etiology/pathophysiology of CH and that improved rates of patient satisfaction can be obtained by directing treatment at R3 or below during ETS or ESB. Applying these findings to the management of craniofacial hyperhidrosis, limiting treatment to an R3 sympathotomy may be sufficient for a large percentage of patients while avoiding the historically high rates of CH seen in this patient population when treated at higher levels, reserving R2 sympathotomy for those patients who fail to achieve satisfactory relief of symptoms from the initial R3 operation.

Endoscopic thoracic sympathectomy continues to offer a definitive treatment of properly selected patients with focal primary hyperhidrosis who have failed nonoperative management. High rates of treatment success in the literature offer similar support for reoperation in patients with primary technical failure or recurrence of symptoms after ETS.

## REFERENCES

1. Lin CC. A new method of thoracoscopic sympathectomy in hyperhidrosis palmaris. Surg Endosc 1990; 4:224–6.
2. Cerfolio RJ, Milanez de Campos JR, Bryant AS, et al. The society of thoracic surgeons expert consensus for the surgical treatment of hyperhidrosis. Ann Thorac Surg 2011;91:1642–8.
3. Chou SH, Kao EL, Lin CC, et al. The importance of classification in sympathetic surgery and a proposed mechanism for compensatory hyperhidrosis: experience with 464 cases. Surg Endosc 2006;20: 1749–53.
4. Yano M, Kiriyama M, Fukai I, et al. Endoscopic thoracic sympathectomy for palmar hyperhidrosis: Efficacy of T2 and T3 ganglion resection. Surgery 2005;138:40–5.
5. Yazbek G, Wolosker N, Kauffman P, et al. Twenty months of evolution following sympathectomy on patients with palmar hyperhidrosis: sympathectomy at the T3 level is better than at the T2 level. Clinics (Sao Paulo) 2009;64:743–9.
6. Lin CC, Telaranta T. Lin-Telaranta classification: the importance of different procedures for different indications in sympathetic surgery. Ann Chir Gynaecol 2001;90:161–6.
7. Ishy A, de Campos JR, Wolosker N, et al. Objective evaluation of patients with palmar hyperhidrosis submitted to two levels of sympathectomy: T3 and T4. Interact Cardiovasc Thorac Surg 2011;12:545–9.
8. Heidemann E, Licht PB. A comparative study of thoracoscopic sympathicotomy versus local surgical treatment for axillary hyperhidrosis. Ann Thorac Surg 2013;95:264–8.
9. Naumann M, Lowe NJ, Kumar CR, et al. Botulinum toxin type a is a safe and effective treatment for axillary hyperhidrosis over 16 months: a prospective study. Arch Dermatol 2003;139:731–6.

10. Lin TS, Chou MC. Needlescopic thoracic sympathetic block by clipping for craniofacial hyperhidrosis. Surg Endosc 2002;16:1055–8.

11. Dewey TM, Herbert MA, Hill SL, et al. One-year follow-up after thoracoscopic sympathectomy for hyperhidrosis: outcomes and consequences. Ann Thorac Surg 2006;81:1227–33.

12. Yang J, Tan JJ, Ye GL, et al. T3/T4 thoracic sympathictomy and compensatory sweating in treatment of palmar hyperhidrosis. Chin Med J (Engl) 2007;120:1574–7.

13. Li X, Tu Y, Lin M, et al. Endoscopic thoracic sympathectomy for palmar hyperhidrosis: a randomized control trial comparing T3 and T2-4 ablation. Ann Thorac Surg 2008;85:1747–52.

14. Weksler B, Blaine G, Souza ZB, et al. Transection of more than one sympathetic chain ganglion for hyperhidrosis increases the severity of compensatory hyperhidrosis and decreases patient satisfaction. J Surg Res 2009;156:110–5.

15. Wait SD, Killory BD, Lekovic GP, et al. Thoracoscopic sympathectomy for hyperhidrosis: analysis of 642 procedures with special attention to Horner's syndrome and compensatory hyperhidrosis. Neurosurgery 2010;67:652–6.

16. Araújo CA, Azevedo IM, Ferreira MA, et al. Compensatory sweating after thoracoscopic sympathectomy: characteristics, prevalence and influence on patient satisfaction. J Bras Pneumol 2009;35:213–20.

17. Murphy MO, Ghosh J, Khwaja N, et al. Upper dorsal endoscopic thoracic sympathectomy: a comparison of one- and two-port ablation techniques. Eur J Cardiothorac Surg 2006;30:223–7.

18. Hsia JY, Chen CY, Hsu CP, et al. Outpatient thoracoscopic limited sympathectomy for hyperhidrosis palmaris. Ann Thorac Surg 1999;67:258–9.

19. Kwong KF, Hobbs JL, Cooper LB, et al. Stratified analysis of clinical outcomes in thoracoscopic sympathectomy for hyperhidrosis. Ann Thorac Surg 2008;85:390–3.

20. Bryant AS, Cerfolio RJ. Satisfaction and compensatory hyperhidrosis rates 5 years and longer after video-assisted thoracoscopic sympathotomy for hyperhidrosis. J Thorac Cardiovasc Surg 2014;147:1160–3.

21. Miller DL, Force SD. Temporary thoracoscopic sympathetic block for hyperhidrosis. Ann Thorac Surg 2008;85(4):1211–4 [discussion 1215–6].

22. Atkinson JLD, Fode-Thomas NC, Fealey RD, et al. Endoscopic transthoracic limited sympathotomy for palmar-plantar hyperhidrosis: outcomes and complications during a 10-year period. Mayo Clin Proc 2011;86:721–9.

23. Zhang B, Li Z, Yang X, et al. Anatomical variations of the upper thoracic sympathetic chain. Clin Anat 2009;22:595–600.

24. Ramsaroop L, Singh B, Moodley J, et al. Anatomical basis for a successful upper limb sympathectomy in the thoracoscopic era. Clin Anat 2004;17:294–9.

25. Chiou TSM, Liao KK. Orientation landmarks of endoscopic transaxillary T-2 sympathectomy for palmar hyperhidrosis. J Neurosurg 1996;85:310–5.

26. Ramsaroop L, Partab P, Singh B, et al. Thoracic origin of a sympathetic supply to the upper limb: the 'nerve of Kuntz' revisited. J Anat 2001;199:675–82.

27. Baumgartner FJ. Thoracoscopic surgery for hyperhidrosis in the presence of congenital azygous lobe and its suspensory web. Tex Heart Inst J 2009;36:44–7.

28. Kauffman P, Wolosker N, de Campos JR, et al. Azygos lobe: a difficulty in video-assisted thoracic sympathectomy. Ann Thorac Surg 2010;89:57–9.

29. Lee SB, Chang JC, Park SQ, et al. Morphometric study of the upper thoracic sympathetic Ganglia. J Korean Neurosurg Soc 2011;50:30–5.

30. Singh B, Moodley J, Ramdial PK. Pitfalls in thoracoscopic sympathectomy: mechanisms for failure. Surg Laparosc Endosc Percutan Tech 2001;11:364–7.

31. de Andrade Filho LO, Kuzniec S, Wolosker N, et al. Technical difficulties and complications of sympathectomy in the treatment of hyperhidrosis: an analysis of 1731 cases. Ann Vasc Surg 2013;27:447–53.

32. Aoki H, Sakai T, Murata H, et al. Extent of sympathectomy affects postoperative compensatory sweating and satisfaction in patients with palmar hyperhidrosis. J Anesth 2014;28:210–3.

33. Baumgartner FJ, Reyes M, Sarkisyan GG, et al. Thoracoscopic sympathicotomy for disabling palmar hyperhidrosis: a prospective randomized comparison between two levels. Ann Thorac Surg 2011;92:2015–9.

34. Kuhajda I, Djuric D, Milos K. Semi-Fowler vs. lateral decubitus position for thoracoscopic sympathectomy in treatment of primary focal hyperhidrosis. J Thorac Dis 2015;7:S5–11.

35. Kuijpers M, Klinkenberg TJ, Bouma W, et al. Single-port one-stage bilateral thoracoscopic sympathicotomy for severe hyperhidrosis: prospective analysis of a standardized approach. J Cardiothorac Surg 2013;8:216–21.

36. Ibrahim M, Allam A. Comparing two methods of thoracoscopic sympathectomy for palmar hyperhidrosis. JAAPA 2014;27:1–4.

37. Li X, Tu YR, Lin M, et al. Minimizing endoscopic thoracic sympathectomy for primary palmar hyperhidrosis: guided by palmar skin temperature and laser doppler blood flow. Ann Thorac Surg 2009;87:427–31.

38. Liu Y, Li H, Zheng X, et al. Sympathicotomy for palmar hyperhidrosis: the association between intraoperative palm temperature change and the

curative effect. Ann Thorac Cardiovasc Surg 2015; 21:359–63.

39. Lin TS. Video-assisted thoracoscopic "resympathicotomy" for palmar hyperhidrosis: analysis of 42 cases. Ann Thorac Surg 2001;72:895–8.

40. Hsu CP, Chen CY, Hsia JY, et al. Resympathectomy for palmar and axillary hyperhidrosis. Br J Surg 1998;85:1504–5.

41. Katara AN, Domino JP, Cheah WK, et al. Comparing T2 and T2–T3 ablation in thoracoscopic sympathectomy for palmar hyperhidrosis: a randomized control trial. Surg Endosc 2007;21:1768–71.

42. Weksler B, Pollice M, Souza ZB, et al. Comparison of ultrasonic scalpel to electrocautery in patients undergoing endoscopic thoracic sympathectomy. Ann Thorac Surg 2009;88:1138–41.

43. Callejas MA, Rubio M, Iglesias M, et al. Video-assisted thoracoscopic sympathectomy for the treatment of facial flushing: ultrasonic scalpel versus diathermy. Arch Bronconeumol 2004;40:17–9.

44. de Campos JRM, Wolosker N, Yazbek G, et al. Comparison of pain severity following video-assisted thoracoscopic sympathectomy: electric versus harmonic scalpels. Interact Cardiovasc Thorac Surg 2010;10:919–22.

45. Kuhajda I, Durić D, Koledin M. Electric vs. harmonic scalpel in treatment of primary focal hyperhidrosis with thoracoscopic sympathectomy. Ann Transl Med 2015;3:211.

46. Lin CC, Mo LR, Lee LS, et al. Thoracoscopic T2-sympathetic block by clipping - a better and reversible operation for treatment of hyperhidrosis palmaris: experience with 326 cases. Eur J Surg Suppl 1998;(580):13–6.

47. Inan K, Goksel OS, Uçak A. Thoracic endoscopic surgery for hyperhidrosis: comparison of different techniques. Thorac Cardiovasc Surg 2008;56:210–3.

48. Coelho Mde S, Silva RF, Mezzalira G, et al. T3T4 endoscopic sympathetic blockade versus T3T4 video thoracoscopic sympathectomy in the treatment of axillary hyperhidrosis. Ann Thorac Surg 2009;88:1780–5.

49. Panhofer P, Ringhofer C, Gleiss A, et al. Quality of life after sympathetic surgery at the T4 ganglion for primary hyperhidrosis: Clip application versus diathermic cut. Int J Surg 2014;12:1478–83.

50. Aydemir B, Imamoglu O, Okay T, et al. Sympathectomy versus Sympathicotomy in Palmar Hyperhidrosis Comparing T3 Ablation. Thorac Cardiovasc Surg 2015;63:715–9.

51. Mohebbi HA, Mehrvarz S, Manoochehry S. Thoracoscopic Sympathicotomy vs Sympathectomy in Primary Hyperhidrosis. Trauma Mon 2012;17:291–5.

52. Scognamillo F, Serventi F, Attene F, et al. T2-T4 sympathectomy versus T3-T4 sympathicotomy for palmar and axillary hyperhidrosis. Clin Auton Res 2011;21:97–102.

53. Hwang JJ, Kim do H, Hong YJ, et al. A comparison between two types of limited sympathetic surgery for palmar hyperhidrosis. Surg Today 2013;43: 397–402.

54. Lee DY, Paik HC, Kim DH, et al. Comparative analysis of T3 selective division of rami communicantes (ramicotomy) to T3 sympathetic clipping in treatment of palmar hyperhidrosis. Clin Auton Res 2003;13:145–7.

55. Kim DH, Paik HC, Lee DY. Comparative analysis of T2 selective division of rami-communicantes (ramicotomy) with T2 sympathetic clipping in the treatment of craniofacial hyperhidrosis. Eur J Cardiothorac Surg 2004;26:396–400.

56. Leseche G, Castier Y, Thabut G, et al. Endoscopic transthoracic sympathectomy for upper limb hyperhidrosis: limited sympathectomy does not reduce postoperative compensatory sweating. J Vasc Surg 2003;37:124–8.

57. Moya J, Ramos R, Morera R, et al. Thoracic sympathicolysis for primary hyperhidrosis: a review of 918 procedures. Surg Endosc 2006;20:598–602.

58. Weksler B, Luketich JD, Shende MR. Endoscopic thoracic sympathectomy: at what level should you perform surgery? Thorac Surg Clin 2008;18:183–91.

59. Kim WO, Kil HK, Yoon KB, et al. Influence of T3 or T4 sympathicotomy for palmar hyperhidrosis. Am J Surg 2010;199:166–9.

60. Abd Ellatif ME, El Hadidi A, Musa AM, et al. Optimal level of sympathectomy for primary palmar Hyperhidrosis: T3 versus T4 in a retrospective Cohort study. Int J Surg 2014;12:778–82.

61. Munia MA, Wolosker N, Kaufmann P, et al. Sustained benefit lasting one year from T4 instead of T3-T4 sympathectomy for isolated axillary hyperhidrosis. Clinics (Sao Paulo) 2008;63:771–4.

62. Guimarães PS, Coelho Mde S, Mendes RG, et al. Ramicotomy in association with endoscopic sympathetic blockade in the treatment of axillary hyperhidrosis. Surg Laparosc Endosc Percutan Tech 2013;23:223–8.

63. Yuncu G, Turk F, Ozturk G, et al. Comparison of only T3 and T3-T4 sympathectomy for axillary hyperhidrosis regarding treatment effect and compensatory sweating. Interact Cardiovasc Thorac Surg 2013;17: 263–7.

64. Bell D, Jedynak J, Bell R. Predictors of outcome following endoscopic thoracic sympathectomy. ANZ J Surg 2014;84:68–72.

65. Nicholas R, Quddus A, Baker DM. Treatment of primary craniofacial hyperhidrosis: a systematic review. Am J Clin Dermatol 2015;16:361–70.

66. Neumayer C, Panhofer P, Jakesz R, et al. Surgical treatment of facial hyperhidrosis and blushing: mid-term results after endoscopic sympathetic block and review of the literature. Eur Surg 2005; 37:127–36.

67. Lin TS, Fang HY, Wu CY. Repeat transthoracic endoscopic sympathectomy for palmar and axillary hyperhidrosis. Surg Endosc 2000;14:134–6.

68. Dumont P, Denoyer A, Robin P. Long-term results of thoracoscopic sympathectomy for hyperhidrosis. Ann Thorac Surg 2004;78:1801–7.

69. Neumayer C, Zacherl J, Holak G, et al. Experience with limited endoscopic thoracic sympathetic block for hyperhidrosis and facial blushing. Clin Auton Res 2003;13:152–7.

70. Licht PB, Clausen A, Ladegaard L. Resympathicotomy. Ann Thorac Surg 2010;89:1087–90.

71. Freeman RK, Van Woerkom JM, Vyverberg A, et al. Reoperative endoscopic sympathectomy for persistent or recurrent palmar hyperhidrosis. Ann Thorac Surg 2009;88:412–6.

# Reversibility of Sympathectomy for Primary Hyperhidrosis

Conor F. Hynes, MD, M. Blair Marshall, MD*

## KEYWORDS

- Primary hyperhidrosis • Endoscopic thoracic sympathectomy • Sympathectomy reversal
- Compensatory sweating • Video-assisted thoracoscopic surgery

## KEY POINTS

- Thoracic sympathetic chain clipping is successfully reversible in most cases when performed early in the postoperative period.
- Histologic studies of sympathetic chains after clipping have found that these nerve bundles regenerate in a progression analogous to peripheral nerve regeneration.
- Insufficient evidence is available to support or refute potential reversibility after a prolonged period of clipping.

## INTRODUCTION

Endoscopic thoracic sympathectomy (ETS) surgery is a highly effective treatment of primary hyperhidrosis (PH) of the palms, face, and axillae that can be performed as an outpatient procedure with low perioperative morbidity. The major adverse effect of the procedure is compensatory sweating (CS), a phenomenon characterized by increased sweating in a dermatomal distribution distal to the level of sympathetic chain clipping. Other less common complaints stimulating desire for reversal include Horner syndrome, bradycardia, gustatory sweating, and excessive dryness of sympathectomized dermatomes.[1]

Reports of clinically significant CS range widely; however, the pathophysiologic mechanism of temperature homeostasis dictates that all patients with normally functioning neural and integumentary systems will experience CS to some degree. A clinically relevant threshold for severity of CS is whether the patient expresses more dissatisfaction with CS postoperatively than with the original symptoms of PH. Reports of this proportion have ranged from of 2% to 13%, with approximately 10% of patients in a temperate climate requesting reversal of ETS if given the option.[1–5] Therefore, it is beneficial to perform ETS in a manner most amenable to reversal. This is the motivation for clipping the sympathetic chain as opposed to cutting it.

Reversal of sympathectomy following clip placement is through their removal via a second outpatient thoracoscopic procedure. Though many surgeons have observed spontaneous nerve regeneration following transection of the sympathetic chain, this approach to sympathectomy generally requires nerve grafting for reversal. Comparisons of sympathetic chain transection to endoscopic clipping have repeatedly found equivalent efficacy for PH symptom control between these techniques.[6] Many surgeons have reported

Disclosure: The authors have received no financial, property or intellectual aid for this research and have no conflicts of interest.
Division of Thoracic Surgery, Georgetown University Hospital, 3800 Reservoir Road Northwest, Washington, DC 20007, USA
* Corresponding author.
E-mail address: conor.f.hynes@gmail.com

1547-4127/16/© 2016 Elsevier Inc. All rights reserved.

thoracic.theclinics.com

good results with clip removal to reverse the symptoms of CS.[1-13] The mechanism of symptom improvement following clip removal is poorly understood; however, results have not been satisfactory for all surgeons. This article focuses on the efficacy of removal of clips as a technique to reverse ETS when the adverse effects outweigh the benefit for patients and underscores factors that can potentially enhance results.

## CLINICAL DATA

Successful reversal has been widely reported following clip removal. Assimilation of data among different surgery groups has been challenging because of substantial variation in clinical application of ETS arising from limitations in the understanding of several pathophysiologic and technical variables. Specific parameters of clip reversal affecting outcome that are not well-defined and, therefore, not standardized include maximal clip duration, projected regeneration interval after clip removal, and optimal clip pressure. Metrics of satisfaction are also difficult to assess with incomplete reporting, lack of universal definitions, and lack of true objective measurements of hyperhidrosis or CS for use across clinical practices. Finally, some concern has arisen regarding a potential placebo effect of unclipping due to paradoxic results of improved CS following reversal without recurrence of PH symptoms, highlighting the subjective nature of both PH and CS.

Most data supporting the reversibility of sympathetic clipping come from small retrospective clinical series. Rates of successful reversal, generally defined as satisfactory improvement of CS, range from 20% to 100% but most often are between 60% and 70%.[1-13] Historically, reporting practices have not always included information regarding clip duration, follow-up intervals, or clip pressure, all of which could impact success.

A commonly held and well-substantiated belief is that earlier clip removal, that is, shorter clip duration, portends a greater likelihood of successful outcome. In theory, this is because inflammatory changes become chronic over extended durations and, eventually, the pathways for nerve regeneration become permanently obliterated. In addition, nerve degeneration and regeneration is a prolonged process, depending on the length of the nerve. Though sympathetic neural transmission is blocked immediately at the time of clip placement, degeneration of the nerve fibers has only just begun. Thus, with early clip removal regeneration is hastened secondary to reduced degeneration. Investigators who have cited their highest reversal success rates at shorter clip

durations indicate optimal clip durations based on findings of 100% reversal after 2 weeks,[10] 78% at 4 weeks,[7] 90% at 8 weeks,[4] 100% at 10 weeks,[1] and 67% to 81% at 6 months.[2,3] Factors such as patient expectations, surgical technique, and follow-up are likely to affect dissimilarity. Unclipping beyond 6 months has resulted in diminishing success rates, providing credence to the proposed theory of maximal clip duration. Yet timing has not always proven to be a strict limitation because successful reversals have been performed at a rate of 50% success after 4 years of clip duration[2] and as long as 4.5 years.[3] These outliers presently have no empirical explanation available but suggest that the premise of a temporal limitation to clipping is an oversimplification of the biomechanics of clipping.

The interval of time to neural recovery after unclipping is also not well defined. Follow-up presents a potent challenge to this question and is perceived to be intimately linked to the physiologic process of nerve degeneration and regeneration initiated by neural crush injury. Because patients with PH often visit surgeons on an as-needed basis and generally stop returning to clinic after reversal, having exhausted surgical therapy, the ultimate patient outcome is sometimes unknown. Months, and perhaps much longer, may be required to regenerate neural tissue,[7] ushering delayed success of reversal in some patients that is not identified at short-term follow-up (see later discussion). Because a standard interval of neural regeneration time has not been delineated, the appropriate follow-up timeframe is unknown. The clinical literature contains many cases of clip removal that achieved satisfactory resolution of CS within a few days to weeks,[9,14] whereas others achieved resolution that was delayed for up to 9 months after clip removal.[9] These contrasting time courses suggest that divergent processes of neural blockade and recovery are taking place in patients with starkly variant recovery intervals.

Another factor obscuring the understanding of reversal outcomes is the matter of unstandardized clip force application. The force of clipping required to inhibit nerve conduction is 30 to 44 g of pressure, whereas commonly used commercial endoclip devices apply 150 g of pressure when executed per the manufacturer specifications.[4] Some surgeons modulate this pressure in an uncontrolled fashion by partially firing the clip; however, this may not be consistently reproducible across cohort of surgeons.[4] The clinical relevance of clip force is considerable because unequal amounts of pressure will result in either simple nerve transmission blockade, crush injury stimulating nerve degeneration while maintaining perineural tissue and structure, or complete nerve transection, each of which have quite disparate clinical consequences. In cases of clinical reversal of clip effect after a span of a few days to a few months,[14,15] it is conceivable that the nerve conduction was simply blocked by the clip without the degree of crush injury required to trigger complete degeneration. In instances when clip removal does not result in CS resolution, excessive clip force may have transected the nerve, resulting in disorganized, and thus ineffective, regeneration.

Perhaps most critical, the psychosocial component of PH cannot be understated. Every aspect of the disease presentation and management is colored by patient idiosyncrasy in this regard, from the level of distress of the primary disease or CS, to degree of overall satisfaction, to the desire for reversal. Moreover, many external factors affect patients differently, hinging on circumstance rather than physiology, including cultural norms, occupational demands, and local climate. Patient satisfaction must be evaluated in the same manner as other subjective measures of health care, such as pain, which are individually assessed. Given that the same propensity for sweating can be distressing in one patient and manageable in another, clinicians must focus on the patient-centered outcome rather than precise physiologic quantities. To this end, an array of scoring systems has been devised to assess distress and treatment satisfaction, and have been used with positive effects. However, these have not been widely adopted; perhaps owing to a perceived need for a clinical threshold rather than a graduated scale.

A well-studied example of the impact of social influence on outcome is demonstrated by research investigating ideal rib level of sympathectomy. Several investigators have identified higher rates of reversal requests following clipping of higher rib levels, as well as lower success of reversal at these levels.[3,12,16] The pathophysiologic mechanism of these differences seems to be multifactorial, with hypotheses involving heightened CS stimulation at these levels and associations with inadvertent blockade of the nearby stellate ganglion. However, central to this issue are the differences in distress stemming from higher perceived visibility of CS at more anatomically superior dermatomes and greater tolerability of imperfect outcomes at more inferior distributions. This distinction is relevant because assumptions about nerve regeneration can easily be confused with psychological results, obfuscating the pursuit and interpretation of neurohistologic evidence.

Aside from the aforementioned inconsistencies surrounding clip reversal, several critics have cited the incongruous relationship between reversal of CS and return of PH symptoms following clip removal,[17–19] suggesting a placebo effect of unclipping. Clinical reviews suggest PH symptoms remain controlled after reversal of CS in up to 42% of cases.[3] The placebo explanation for this sporadic observation is currently unproven but certainly plausible. Yet, granted that the success of ETS and of its reversal is primarily founded on the subjective patient perception of symptoms, clinicians can reasonably consider this phenomenon to be beneficial to the patient. Furthermore, this is by no means a universal finding and does not exclude other contributing factors. Indeed, many surgeons have reported a concordant return of PH symptoms along with resolution of CS.[1,2,4,5,7,9–11]

In opposition to the placebo interpretation, clinicians must also consider that the generation of neural pathways defining CS is based on observation rather than biochemical evidence. Therefore, clinicians cannot assume that resolution of CS symptoms and re-emergence of PH symptoms will occur in perfect symmetry because these pathways may be quite different. It is equally plausible that following neural crush injury sympathetic innervation of blocked dermatomes returns to an attenuated degree in the same way that other soft tissue injuries recover only 80% of their original integrity. Other neuroscientific research supports a mechanism of interruption of negative feedback signaling from the autonomic nervous system to the hypothalamus caused by clipping that produces unrestricted positive afferent signals to the inferior sweat glands.[20] Ultimately, more data on this topic are needed.

## HISTOLOGY

The theoretic basis of sympathetic chain regeneration is primarily extrapolated from general principles of peripheral nerve regeneration coupled with clinical findings. Unlike nerve transection, a crush injury that preserves the perineural sheath maintains a pathway for regrowth of the nerve fibers along its original course. Initially, following this type of nerve injury, the process of Wallerian degeneration advances over approximately 6 to 8 weeks.[21] Once debris from compromised nerve components has been eliminated, subsequent regeneration then takes place over a span of months.[22]

A paucity of confirmatory histologic data has been collected under controlled settings to characterize the effects of surgical clipping of the sympathetic chain. In recent years, 4 small series using applied animal models have been designed to evaluate these effects while using the contralateral chain as the unclipped control comparison. Each used different time intervals and different species; however, taken together, these offer some clarification of the mechanism of clipping and its reversibility.

A porcine model devised by Loscertales and colleagues,[23] published in 2012, examined the nerves after 10-day and 20-day intervals of clipping. This study identified clear evidence of Wallerian degeneration during the expected range of the first month after crush injury, including macrophage phagocytosis of myelin debris. Furthermore, it confirmed that the injury of the clips did preserve the structural morphology of nerves, which would later serve as the scaffolding for the regenerative process.

During the same year, Candas and colleagues[24] used a leporine model to clip chains for 48 hours, then unclip and biopsy immediately and after 45 days. Early inflammatory cell infiltration was again identified at 48 hours. Confirmation of Wallerian degeneration was shown at 45 days, with no signs of regeneration at this point. Although not contradictory to the theory of peripheral nerve regeneration, the investigators raised the logical point that nerve fragility could have affected the results. In addition to leporine sympathetic chains being smaller than human homologs, they reported use of clip pressures averaging 150 g, well in excess of that required to block signal transmission even in the larger, more durable nerves of humans. Implicitly, clinicians understand that some degree of nerve pressure crosses the upper limit of crush injury into frank transection. Thus, a matter of concern that deserves further regulation is the application of ETS is clip pressure.

These studies were followed by an ovine study performed by Thomsen and colleagues[17] that clipped chains for 7 days, and biopsied at intervals of 4 weeks and 12 weeks after unclipping. Findings at 4 weeks were again congruent with expected degeneration, with decreased myelinating cells and number of synapses. At 12 weeks, Schwann cell morphology had returned to normal and the number of synapses had again increased. At both intervals the neurofilament proteins were similar between clipped chains and unclipped controls, demonstrating that an appropriate level of crush injury pressure had been used to maintain neural structures that allowed for regeneration.

Finally, the hircine model used by Erol and colleagues[25] clipped chains for 4 weeks and biopsied immediately, as well as at 4 weeks after unclipping. The immediate biopsies show expected degeneration. At the 4-week interval, biopsies showed reaccumulation of Schwann cells, suggesting reconstitution of myelin was occurring.

Though these models provide limited snapshots of the process of nerve degeneration and regeneration, they all support the same theoretic progression, analogous to peripheral nerves. Combined with clinical findings of resolution of CS symptoms, these results offer highly convincing support to the hypothesis that nerve regeneration plays an important role in CS reversal.

## DISCUSSION

The thoracic surgery community has made great strides to enhance the standardization of ETS indications and technique, as well as to promote evidence-based practices regarding reversal of clipping. The official statement by the Society of Thoracic Surgeons has expressed an appropriate level of apprehension toward recommending reversal due to inconsistent outcomes.[26] Undoubtedly, the current status of the surgical management of PH calls for a greater degree of standardization of ETS and reversal, including the technique of sympathetic chain clipping; the indication for reversal; and recommendations for intervals of clip duration and unclipping follow-up that would allow a high likelihood of a positive outcome. Yet the high rates of intolerable CS, the multitude of reported effective clip reversals, and the lack of effective alternative management for CS support the use of clipping instead of nerve transection specifically to allow for the possibility of reversal. The corollary to this recommendation is that patients must be quoted a reasonable expected rate of successful reversal before undergoing ETS based on accurate local institutional outcomes or from the general body of thoracic surgery literature.

Several specific areas of further investigation thus have emerged that are very likely to enhance clip reversal outcomes. Additional animal models need to be performed to delineate effects of clipping over a range of pressures between 30 g and 150 g to elucidate whether reversal rates can be improved without sacrificing current high efficacy, thereby establishing a new benchmark. Subsequent enhancements of clip device design could then follow and be disseminated. A clinically meaningful designation for CS, such as "intolerable CS" that is defined as severity warranting surgical reversal, must be promulgated to eliminate confusion surrounding the rates and relevance of CS following ETS. A clip duration must be agreed on that offers a reasonably high likelihood of effective reversal, with unclipping beyond that duration carrying a weaker recommendation. This duration would likely directly depend on the standard clip pressure used. Finally, to ascertain true reversal rates, continued study must establish the expected interval across which a positive result is likely to occur in order to prescribe the necessary follow-up interval for patients awaiting the effects of reversal.

At this time, clinicians do not have objective data to demonstrate the mechanism of CS reversal and return-to-normal dermatomal distribution of sweat gland activity. In fact, clinicians do not know whether unclipping causes resolution of CS symptoms by a process of normalization of nerve conduction pathways at all. These undefined neural regenerative pathways could explain why some patients have resolution of CS without return of PH symptoms. Given that this theory is the cornerstone of the therapeutic effect of ETS clip reversal, further study is required.

PH is a complex disease process that is not addressed simply by an outpatient sympathetic chain interruption. Extensive patient counseling and initial attempts at nonoperative management of symptoms are widely supported by the thoracic surgery community. On arrival at the decision to proceed with surgical management, clinicians must accept and prepare for the possibility that a significant proportion of patients will be dissatisfied with the adverse effects. The current lack of understanding of the neurochemical basis of sympathetic chain injury and regeneration demands further study. However, given the large body of reproducible evidence demonstrating that unclipping the sympathetic chain results in improved patient satisfaction in most cases, the authors' recommendation at this time is to consider ETS by clipping a potentially reversible procedure when CS symptoms are intolerable.

## REFERENCES

1. Hynes CF, Yamaguchi S, Bond CD, et al. Reversal of sympathetic interruption by removal of clips. Ann Thorac Surg 2015;99:1020–4.
2. Reisfeld R. Sympathectomy for hyperhidrosis: should we place the clamps at T2-T3 or T3-T4? Clin Auton Res 2006;16:384–9.
3. Sugimura H, Spratt EH, Compeau CG, et al. Thoracoscopic sympathetic clipping for hyperhidrosis: long-term results and reversibility. J Thorac Cardiovasc Surg 2009;137:1370–8.
4. Kang CW, Choi SY, Moon SW, et al. Short-term and intermediate-term results after unclipping. Surg Laparosc Endosc Percutan Tech 2008;18:469–73.
5. Chou SH, Kao EL, Lin CC, et al. The importance of classification in sympathetic surgery and a proposed mechanism for compensatory hyperhidrosis: experience with 464 cases. Surg Endosc 2006;20:1749–53.
6. Kocher GJ, Taha A, Ahler M, et al. Is clipping the preferable technique to perform sympathicotomy? A retrospective study and review of the literature. Langenbecks Arch Surg 2015;400:107–12.
7. Jo KH, Moon SW, Kim YD, et al. New protocol for a reversal operation in endoscopic thoracic sympathetic clamping: pulling back the suture sling clinked to the clip under local anesthesia. Surg Laparosc Endosc Percutan Tech 2007;17:29–32.
8. Balsalobre RM, Mata NM, Izquierdo RR, et al. Guidelines on surgery of the thoracic sympathetic nervous system. Arch Bronconeumol 2010;47:94–102.
9. Lin CC, Mo LR, Lee LS, et al. Thoracoscopic T2-sympathetic block by clipping–a better and reversible operation for treatment of hyperhidrosis palmaris: experience with 326 cases. Eur J Surg Suppl 1998;580:13–6.
10. Lin TS, Chou MC. Treatment of palmar hyperhidrosis using needlescopic T2 sympathetic block by clipping: analysis of 102 cases. Int Surg 2004;89:198–201.
11. Lin TS. Endoscopic clipping in video-assisted thoracoscopic sympathetic blockade for axillary hyperhidrosis. Surg Endosc 2001;15:126–8.
12. Reisfeld R. One-year follow-up after thoracoscopic sympathectomy for hyperhidrosis. Ann Thorac Surg 2007;83:358–9.
13. Krasna MJ. Thoracoscopic sympathectomy. Thorac Surg Clin 2010;20:323–30.
14. Dumont P. Side effects and complications of surgery for hyperhidrosis. Thorac Surg Clin 2008;18(2):18193–207.
15. Miller DL, Force SD. Outpatient microthoracoscopic sympathectomy for palmar hyperhidrosis. Ann Thorac Surg 2007;83:1850–3.
16. Dewey TM, Hebert MA, Hill SL, et al. One-year follow-up after thoracoscopic sympathectomy for hyperhidrosis. Ann Thorac Surg 2006;81:1227–33.
17. Thomsen LL, Mikkelsen RT, Derejko M, et al. Sympathetic block by metal clips may be a reversible operation. Interact Cardiovasc Thorac Surg 2014;19:908–13.
18. Schick CH, Bischof G, Cameron AAEP, et al. Sympathetic chain clipping for hyperhidrosis is not a reversible procedure. Surg Endosc 2013;27:3043.
19. Licht PB. Invited commentary. Ann Thorac Surg 2015;99:1020–4.
20. Loewy AD, Spyer KM. Central regulation of autonomic functions. New York: Oxford University Press; 1990. p. 88–103.
21. Menorca RMG, Fussell TS, Elfar JC. Nerve physiology: mechanisms of injury and recovery. Hand Clin 2013;29:317–30.

22. Burnett MG, Zager EL. Pathophysiology of peripheral nerve injury: a brief review. Neurosurg Focus 2004;15:1.

23. Loscertales J, Congregado M, Jimenez-Merchan R, et al. Sympathetic chain clipping for hyperhidrosis is not a reversible procedure. Surg Endosc 2012;26:1258–63.

24. Candas F, Gorur R, Hahlolu A, et al. The effects of clipping on thoracic sympathetic nerve in rabbits: early and late histopathological findings. Thorac Cardiovasc Surg 2012;60:280–4.

25. Erol MM, Salci K, Melek H, et al. Can thoracic sympathetic nerve damage be reversed? Thorac Cardiovasc Surg 2014;63:720–2.

26. Cerfolio RJ, de Campos JRM, Bryant AS, et al. The society of Thoracic Surgeons expert consensus for the surgical treatment of hyperhidrosis. Ann Thorac Surg 2011;91:1642–8.

# Reconstruction of the Sympathetic Chain

Cliff P. Connery, MD

## KEYWORDS

- Video-assisted thoracic sympathectomy • Da Vinci robot • Nerve reconstruction
- Interposition graft

## KEY POINTS

- Sympathectomy for hyperhidrosis despite proper patient selection and surgical techniques can occasionally result in adverse side effects that cause the patient to regret surgery and request reversal.
- Sympathetic nerve regeneration and symptom reversal has been described in experimental and clinical series by various nerve grafting techniques.
- Use of the da Vinci robot allows sympathetic nerve interposition grafting to most closely mirror the principles of peripheral nerve reconstruction.
- Robotic device features of high magnification, scaling of movement, and distally articulated micro-instrumentation facilitates minimally invasive dissection and suturing any nerve graft interposition.
- Use of standardized quality of life assessment tools, physiologic measurements, and long-term follow-up is needed to better compare results of different reconstruction techniques.

 Video content accompanies this article at http://www.thoracic.theclinics.com.

## NERVE RECONSTRUCTION

Video-assisted thoracic sympathectomy is the treatment of choice for patients with severe palmar and axillary hyperhidrosis that has been refractory to conservative treatments. The immediate success rates for control of primary palmar symptoms are greater than 98%.[1] Many patients experience some side effects, such as compensatory sweating, excessive dryness, mild reduction of heart rate, and heat intolerance, but on balance are satisfied with the procedure and have a sustained improvement in quality of life.[2] Severe side effects or complications that make patients regret having had the operation and wish for reversal are rare.[3,4] However, given the prevalence of severe focal hyperhidrosis estimated as 2.8% of the US population,[5] there is a discrete subset of patients whose quality of life is significantly impacted by side effects or complications

after sympathetic surgery that they regret the procedure and wish they could have their surgery reversed. It should be noted that in patients with craniofacial hyperhidrosis or facial blushing, the success and satisfaction rates are a bit less than that of patients who have had surgery for palmar and axillary sweating.[6]

Sympathectomy has been performed by a variety of techniques, such as resection of the chain and ganglion, sympathicotomy or transection of the chain sharply or with energy devices, interruption of the rami of the ganglion, and clip interruption. The theory behind the clipping procedure[7] is that clip compression of the nerve can provide symptomatic efficacy but provide a potentially reversible procedure if a patient develops severe intolerable side effects. This has been evaluated in experimental and clinical models. Although there have been some groups reporting reversal

Dyson Center, Thoracic Oncology, Vassar Brothers Medical Center, 3rd Floor, 45 Reade Place, Poughkeepsie, NY 12601, USA
E-mail address: cconnery@health-quest.org

Thorac Surg Clin 26 (2016) 427–434
http://dx.doi.org/10.1016/j.thorsurg.2016.06.007
1547-4127/16/© 2016 Elsevier Inc. All rights reserved.

of adverse symptoms with clip removal, clearly it does not work in all patients.[8,9]

There have been significant discussions in the literature and at scientific meetings as to methods to try to minimize the dissatisfaction with sympathetic surgery by improving patient selection and modifying surgical techniques, which it is hoped will result in a lower number of patients with important side effects. A crucial part of patient selection is ensuring that patients have had a proper trial of conservative methods. Although controversial,[10] avoiding T2 ganglion interruption and limiting the number of levels divided have been proposed as strategies to reduce compensatory sweating by the Society of Thoracic Surgeons Consensus and other groups.[1,11] Despite all of these efforts, there still is a patient population for which the severe side effects, most commonly compensatory sweating, remain the significant impediment to patient quality of life. It is for that reason that direct means of reversal with nerve grafting has been explored and used clinically in several centers.

## NERVE REGENERATION

Most large series show some patients who have developed delayed recurrent symptoms believed to be caused by spontaneous nerve regeneration. It is postulated that in these situations the transected nerves develop sprouting and if the transected ends remain in proximity, the nerve can spontaneously regenerate. It is for this reason that many surgeons who use sympathicotomy take care to separate the transected ends of the nerve root to try to limit that recurrence.

Peripheral nerve graft reconstruction is an established technique to allow regeneration of injured somatic nerves. The method of regeneration includes the sprouting of nerve buds from the proximal end of a transected nerve, which then traverses a conduit to connect to the distal transected nerve. There are certain chemotactic factors presumed to help this process occur. Conduits have usually been interposition grafts of autologous nerves or more recently irradiated allografts. Synthetic collagen tubes are available for short segment graft reconstruction. These principles of peripheral nerve graft have been applied to the reconstruction of sympathetic nerve in experimental and clinical series.[12–14]

## EXPERIMENTAL SYMPATHETIC NERVE GRAFT RECONSTRUCTION

There have been several investigators who have used animal models to test the concept of sympathetic nerve regeneration by grafting. In 1981 Purves and coworkers[15] reported the reinnervation of autotransplanted sympathetic ganglia in a guinea pig survival model. Matsumoto and coworkers[16] used conduits made of chitosan tubes to reconstruct a resected segment of upper thoracic sympathetic chain in dogs by suturing the tube as an interposition conduit between the severed nerve edges at thoracotomy in a survival study. Nerve ingrowth was seen at 3 months. Observation of improvement of Horner syndrome and foreleg temperature was noted in the subsequent animals that were sacrificed at 7 and 12 months. Necropsy demonstrated histologic confirmation of regeneration.

Our group evaluated the technical feasibility of a minimally invasive da Vinci robotic-assisted procedure to reconstruct the thoracic sympathetic chain using interposition autologous nerve graft and direct suture with 10–0 nylon. We believed that the technical advantages of a da Vinci robotic approach allowed nerve reconstruction to be done in a minimally invasive thoracoscopic approach. The characteristics of the robot that are ideally situated for performing a microsurgical procedure include:

- High-magnification
- Three-dimensional optics
- Scaling of motion
- Distal articulation
- Microinstrumentation

The feasibility of this technique was tested in a nonsurvival model where it was proven that the robotic-assisted technique did allow for a technically facile sutured nerve anastomosis and that the intercostal nerve as opposed to the sural nerve was a better size match to use as a nerve conduit in the pig.[17] A pig autologous sympathetic nerve reconstruction survival model was subsequently developed. Using a thoracoscopic, minimally invasive approach with the Standard daVinci Robot (Intuitive Surgical, Sunnyvale, CA) a representative segment of thoracic sympathetic chain was resected, and a nearby intercostal nerve was harvested and sutured to the sympathetic chain using interrupted 10–0 nylon sutures on the epineurium, which mirrors the approach of a standard peripheral nerve graft reconstruction. At sacrifice 6 months later, the reconstructed nerve was viable and showed nerve regeneration by light microscopy and electron microscopy.[18]

## CLINICAL EXPERIENCE WITH SYMPATHETIC NERVE RECONSTRUCTION

In 1998, Telaranta[19] reported the results of a unilateral sympathetic nerve reconstruction using open thoracotomy and sural nerve graft with 9–0 nylon and fibrin glue as an interposition graft in a patient who had had previous sympathectomy and had intolerable symptoms of exercise intolerance and compensatory sweating. At 1 year, the patient had unilateral recurrence of sweating in the anhidrotic areas, decrease of compensatory sweating to tolerable levels, and the ability to exercise in the heat. This investigator had continued clinical activity with nerve reconstruction using a videothoracoscopic approach, autologous intercostal nerve transposition, and a fibrin glue anastomosis.[20] A recent paper[21] evaluated the long-term outcomes of 19 of the 150 patients who had undergone sympathetic nerve reconstruction by this group. Essentially 75% of these patients had experienced improvement with 50% of the patients reporting a remarkable benefit. Unfortunately, because of lack of record availability at older clinics and inadequate contact information they did not have data on more of their patients. It should be noted that 11% of their patients who underwent planned nerve reconstruction could not have the procedure completed because of technical factors. Problems cited included extensive adhesions, more than three ganglia destroyed at the original surgery, and inadequate interposition graft length.

One of the larger published series was that of Haam and colleagues[22] who performed sympathetic nerve reconstruction using autologous intercostal nerve for patients with severe compensatory sweating after sympathectomy. Nine of 19 patients operated on through a thoracoscopic technique had improvement. Three patients had marked improvement, in six the improvement was characterized as mild, there were eight patients without improvement, and two were lost to follow-up. Review of their paper shows that this neurologic anastomosis was an end-to-side intercostal to sympathetic chain graft with fibrin glue. The author stated that direct suture would require a thoracotomy and made this modified approach to be able to offer a thoracoscopic solution to reconstruction for these patients.

There have been other case reports of nerve graft with fibrin glue anastomosis.[23] Another approach was reported by the Melbourne group using an autologous superficial arm vein as the conduit with thoracoscopic interposition, the anastomosis being constructed with fibrin glue. In these two patients, there was long-term follow-up at 5 and 8 years showing a moderate improvement in quality of life in one and the other patient having a mild positive effect on quality of life. The attractiveness of this procedure is that it increases the availability of autologous conduit

material and reduces the likelihood of donor site deficits.[24]

We used our previously described animal experimental experience with da Vinci robotic nerve grafting for our first clinical case, which was reported at the International Symposium on Sympathetic Surgery in Odense.[25] The approach for our clinical series is described next.

## SYMPATHETIC NERVE RECONSTRUCTION
### Preoperative Planning

A standard history and physical is performed as part of preoperative planning. It is important to review the initial symptoms that the patient had before sympathectomy and to review the surgical procedure that was done to try to treat the symptom complex.

- Current complaints (eg, compensatory sweating)
- Distribution of the affected area
- Patient's exercise capacity
- Resting heart rate
- The ability to increase the heart rate with exercise
- Heat intolerance

On physical examination, it is important to document any findings of Horner syndrome, the moisture distribution of the patient, and relative temperature of the extremities. For those patients with exercise limitation, an exercise limited cardiac stress test should be performed and if available pre-exercise and postexercise thermographic camera imaging can be performed to look at temperature distribution of the patient. If a patient does not demonstrate evidence of severe compensatory sweating when examined in the office, it is recommended that the patient submit photographic documentation of the usual pattern of their sweat when they are distressed by it.

There are other more rare complications that were anecdotally reported with hyperhidrosis surgery, which should be noted and documented. For example, hypopigmentation, intercostal neuralgia, and such complications as Horner syndrome.[26]

Quality of life assessment should be done with specific standardized forms, such as the Dermatology Life Quality Index,[27] Short Form-36,[28–30] and the quality assessment tools of Milanez de Campos and colleagues[2] as recommended by the International Society of Sympathetic Surgery.

### Plan for Reconstruction

It is important to accurately estimate the extent to which the sympathetic chain has been interrupted and also to understand the technique that was used to interrupt the chain. It is likely that thermal ablation–type techniques may have more extensive destruction of the chain and require a longer segment of interposition graft. To identify or estimate the amount of chain that was interrupted it is crucial to review the patient's operative report and any available imaging if possible. It should be remembered that there has been nonstandard nomenclature used in reports and the literature to describe the anatomic aspects of surgical procedures on the sympathetic chain. This hopefully has been rectified by the recommendation of the Society of Thoracic Surgeons consensus statement on the treatment of hyperhidrosis, which recommends using a rib-based nomenclature system to describe the level of nerve interruption.[1] However, if there is a question from the operative report as to what was described, it is recommended that a discussion with the original operating surgeon be carried out to get a better understanding of the extent of chain disruption.

Available imaging should be obtained and reviewed for locations of clips and to identify whether or not there is extensive pleural thickening or some other factors that might limit the procedure being done in a minimally invasive approach. When this is done, an estimate as to the length of conduit needed can be generated. The options to discuss with the patient are using autologous intercostal nerve, sural nerve, or a synthetic biodegradable conduit. This synthetic conduit probably should be used only for short-segment interruptions. Although processed allografts are available, the need for immunosuppression would not likely make its use for this indication warranted.[12,13]

If intercostal nerve is chosen, the planned harvest should be below the level of the fourth rib so that the hoped for regeneration of the sympathetic chain can travel with intercostal nerves in the upper thorax and allow reinnervation of the anhidrotic areas of the chest.

Informed consent discussion should outline the outcomes that would occur if there was a complete reversal. This would theoretically result in a recurrence of the original symptoms that the patient had complained of before sympathectomy and a reduction in the untoward side effects, such as compensatory sweating, anhidrosis, and if present, bradycardia. However, it is unclear whether or not a full reversal will occur or even a partial reversal. The potential patient should be aware that it is possible that they will have no benefit from the surgery but still be subject to the risks associated with thoracic surgery. The general risks are intercostal neuralgia from incisions in the intercostal space, a small chance for bleeding,

adhesions of the lung to the parietal pleura, and an air leak that could require longer chest tube drainage time.

In particular for this operation, the risks include the possibility of further injury to the sympathetic chain and specifically Horner syndrome, which may not have developed initially. Many of the patients who request reversal have had interruption at the level of the second rib, which at the time of nerve reconstruction surgery requires "freshening up" of the proximal nerve just below the stellate ganglion. It is possible that traction injury or direct injury to the stellate ganglion could occur, which could result in either a temporary or permanent component of Horner syndrome.

In addition, the risks of complications from nerve graft harvest should be delineated. These are different depending on the autologous graft. Sural nerve results in anesthesia of the lateral aspect of the lower leg and foot or possible wound complications in the lower extremity. Use of the intercostal nerve results in an area of numbness or possibly intercostal neuralgia, and burning discomfort in the chest, which may be permanent and should be considered.

It should be emphasized that in this operation there is the possibility of no benefit and further injury.

### Preparation and Patient Positioning

The patient is anesthetized with double-lumen tube placement and placed in the lateral decubitus position; we do not use a bean bag. The patient is sterilely prepared and draped and the lower leg is prepared and draped if sural nerve harvest is planned. The sural nerve is not harvested until the exploration is carried out, the sympathetic chain identified, and estimates of needed graft length performed.

When using the da Vinci robotic SI System (Intuitive Surgical, Sunnyvale, CA), the robot is docked from above the patient's head, and given some of the obstruction to ready bedside access that occurs in that situation, we use a clear plastic sterile drape as part of our drape for the patient, over the head, so that the anesthesiologist has better visibility of the double-lumen tube and access in this cramped location.

### Port Placement

For the SI device, the ports are placed in a configuration similar to that used for a totally portal robotic lobectomy as described by Cerfolio.[29] A 12-mm port is used for the camera port; robotic 8-mm ports for the left hand and right-handed port; and an assistant port inferior to the anterior port and the camera port to allow passage of sutures, graft material, suctioning, and other assistant activities. With the SI device, there is an additional port that is available for retraction if necessary. Because these patients have had prior thoracic surgery, our initial port placement is performed with a 5-mm thoracoscopic camera and a 5-mm optical trocar technique to ensure that we have free space and avoid injury on entry into the thorax. This scope is then used to direct placement of the other robotic ports. The optical port is then "up sized" to a standard cannula for the procedure (**Fig. 1**).

### The Robot Is then Docked

Intrathoracic adhesions if present in the superior thorax are mobilized to allow exposure of the upper thoracic chain. For those patients who need intercostal nerve graft interposition, the exposure has to allow for harvesting of an appropriate length of intercostal nerve. Therefore, any adhesions that would preclude that are also lysed.

The area of the sympathetic chain is identified. The scarred ends of the chain proximally and distally are redivided sharply with the Potts scissors (Intuitive Surgical) and the nerve fascicles are identified. Then, using microinstrumentation with black diamond forceps and Potts scissors (Intuitive Surgical), dissect the sympathetic chain to provide a proper edge for grafting. It should be remembered that the area of nerve injury can extend away from the scarred end. It is recommended to "bread loaf" the nerve until more normal structure is identified.[12] No energy is used on the nerve. Any bleeding away from the nerve is controlled with bipolar cautery to avoid transmission of that energy and further injury. Care is particularly taken with the dissection,

cephalad in the vicinity of the stellate ganglion. Mobilization and traction on the stellate ganglion is avoided.

When we have thus identified nerve proximally and distally, the autologous graft is harvested. Our practice is to start with the distal anastomosis first, which is done with 8–0 monofilament sutures placed through the epineurium of the freshened-up sympathetic chain and the interposition graft (**Fig. 2**, Video 1). The interposition graft is then trimmed to the appropriate length to allow direct suturing of the graft to the proximal end (**Fig. 3**). This creates a tension-free anastomosis. Hemostasis is ensured and the remaining graft is then retrieved to use in the contralateral side.

If there is available pleura, a flap is mobilized to place over the graft to try to minimize any disruption with movement of the lung. A chest tube is placed through the thoracostomy, the lung is reinflated under vision with the scope, and the wounds are closed. The patient is then repositioned on the contralateral side for reconstruction of that side. A multicostal intercostal nerve block is done before reinflating the lung.

At the conclusion of the procedure, the patient is extubated, brought to the postsurgical recovery area, and given additional analgesics as necessary. Chest radiograph is performed to verify satisfactory expansion of the lung. The chest tubes are removed when air leak has ceased and drainage is appropriate. The patient is discharged on oral analgesics.

## RESULTS

Our group reported the medium-term follow-up of our first three patients who had undergone sympathetic nerve graft reconstruction using the da Vinci

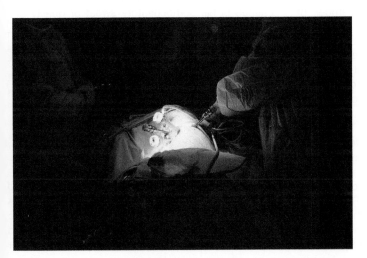

**Fig. 1.** Port placement for da Vinci robotic-assisted sympathetic nerve reconstruction.

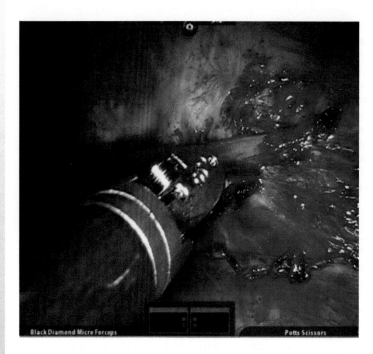

**Fig. 2.** Distal nerve anastomosis.

robotic approach and direct suture. This was reported at the 2015 International Symposium on Sympathetic Surgery meeting.[30] A summary of the cases follows.

A 46-year-old man with craniofacial palmar and axillary sweat had undergone sympathectomy at R2, R3, R4, and R5 at another institution in April of 2010. He complained of fatigue, inability to raise his heart rate, and severe compensatory sweating. His heart rate was in the upper 40s to low 50s. At the time of surgery, we identified what appeared to be a graftable intervening ganglia on each side. We therefore had two discrete interposition grafts on each side. Nerve graft reconstruction using intercostal nerve grafts and direct 8–0 monofilament suture was performed in September of 2010. He had significant improvement in heart rate and exercise capacity starting after 4 months from the surgery. The return of sweating in his anhidrotic upper thoracic areas and moderate reduction in compensatory sweating took longer. He had sweat return to his upper thorax, arms, and neck, but not to his head. Overall, his quality of life was significantly improved. This was measured by Short Form-36 and Dermatology Life Quality Index (Courtesy of Dr Finlay).

The second patient, who had complaints of severe compensatory sweating and exercise intolerance after undergoing an R2, R3, and R4 sympathicotomy, and redo sympathectomy in 2007 for persistent symptoms, had resting heart rate of 44 and a stress test of 71% of predicted that required dobutamine to get a satisfactory exercise component. He had a significant improvement in heart rate and exercise capacity; compensatory sweating moderately improved; and he had sweat return to the axilla, upper extremities, and face with exercise. His quality of life is mildly improved.

The third patient, who had severe compensatory sweating and no cardiac complaints after undergoing an R2 and R3 sympathectomy for craniofacial and palmar sweat, had severe compensatory sweating and heat intolerance, but no other cardiac limitations. He underwent sural nerve graft reconstruction in April of 2013, and has had a mild improvement in sweating, but no significant change in his compensatory sweat or quality of life at this point in time.

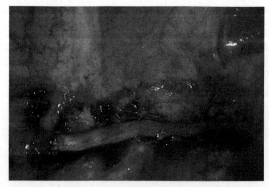

**Fig. 3.** Completed sutured nerve interposition graft.

**Table 1**
**Results October 2015**

| DOS | Heart Rate | Exercise | CS | Sweat Return | Quality of Life |
|---|---|---|---|---|---|
| September 2010 | +++ | +++ | Very improved | ++ | +++ |
| December 2011 | ++ | ++ | Moderately improved | ++ | + |
| April 2013 | = | = | No change | + | No change |

*Abbreviations:* CS, compensatory sweating; DOS, date of surgery.

Tabular results are as noted. In this group of patients, mean postoperative length of stay was 1.3 days, and chest tube duration was 1 day. There were no complications (**Table 1**).

## SUMMARY

Sympathetic nerve regeneration has been proven in experimental models and clinically. Patients with severe side effects or complications from sympathectomy for hyperhidrosis who have exhausted the limited options for treatment should be offered nerve graft reconstruction as an opportunity for them to be able to reverse these adverse symptoms and to have measurable improvements in their quality of life.

The da Vinci robotic nerve graft reconstruction provides a platform for effecting this nerve reconstruction using a minimally invasive technique. It provides excellent visualization, dissection, and neurolysis under high magnification with microsurgical instruments and allows performance of a standard nerve graft reconstruction, whether that be with autologous intercostal or sural nerve or theoretically with the use of commercially available synthetic tubes.

Although a nerve interposition can be glued in place with biologic glue as described by other authors, this procedure does not mirror what are clinically accepted principles for peripheral nerve surgery. Indeed, if one is to undertake nerve reconstruction, eliminating other variables, such as inadequate neurolysis or nonstandard anastomosis, should be paramount in the planning of the procedure.

There remain several questions and it is hoped that increased clinical experience will provide some guidance.

- Does the time from initial surgery have a major impact on outcomes?
- Should clips routinely be removed and the patient observed for recovery even if many years from initial clip placement?
- Does the presence or absence of ganglia impact results?
- Are collagen conduits and other synthetics acceptable?

In the future, it is possible that the nerve reconstruction can be augmented with stem cells or other growth factors. Newer iterations of the robotic device, such as the currently used da Vinci Xi device, allows the use of smaller ports, facilitates setup, and may provide an additional advantage. There are limited options for patients with severe compensatory sweating that has not responded to conservative measures. If the quality of life is significantly impaired and the patient is properly counseled, sympathetic nerve reconstruction is a reasonable option to try to improve quality of life.

## ACKNOWLEDGMENTS

The collaboration of Scott Belsley, MD, and Noel Perin, MD, in our experimental and clinical series was invaluable.

## SUPPLEMENTARY DATA

Supplementary data related to this article can be found at http://dx.doi.org/10.1016/j.thorsurg.2016. 06.007.

## REFERENCES

1. Cerfolio RJ, Milanez de Campos JR, Bryant AS, et al. The Society of Thoracic Surgeons expert consensus for the surgical treatment of hyperhidrosis. Ann Thorac Surg 2011;91:1642–8.
2. Milanez de Campos JR, Kauffman P, Werebe EC, et al. Quality of life before and after thoracic sympathectomy: report on 378 operated patients. Ann Thorac Surg 2003;76:886–91.
3. Chwajol M, Barrenechea IJ, Chakraborty S, et al. Impact of compensatory hyperhidrosis on patient satisfaction after endoscopic thoracic sympathectomy. Neurosurgery 2009;64:511–8.
4. Bryant AS, Cerfolio RJ. Satisfaction and compensatory hyperhidrosis rates 5 years and longer after video-assisted thoracoscopic sympathotomy for hyperhidrosis. J Thorac Cardiovasc Surg 2014;147: 1160–3.
5. Strutton DR, Kowalski JW, Glaser DA, et al. US prevalence of hyperhidrosis and impact on individuals

with axillary hyperhidrosis: results from a national survey. J Am Acad Dermatol 2004;51:241–8.

6. Licht PB, Ladegaard L, Pilegaard HK. Thoracoscopic sympathectomy for isolated facial blushing. Ann Thorac Surg 2006;11:59–62.

7. Lin CC, Mo LR, Lee LS, et al. Thoracoscopic T2 – sympathetic block by clipping: a better and reversible operation for treatment of hyperhidrosis palmaris: experience with 326 cases. Eur J Surg 1998; 580:13–6.

8. Hynes CF, Yamaguchi S, Bond CD, et al. Reversal of sympathetic interruption by removal of clips. Ann Thorac Surg 2015;99:1020–4.

9. Sugimura H, Spratt EH, Compeau CG, et al. Thoracoscopic sympathetic clipping for hyperhidrosis: long-term results and reversibility. J Thorac Cardiovasc Surg 2009;137:1370–8.

10. Kopelman D, Hashmonai M. The correlation between the method of sympathetic ablation for palmar hyperhidrosis and the occurrence of compensatory hyperhidrosis: a review. World J Surg 2008;32: 2343–56.

11. Balsalobre RM, Mata NM, Izquierdo RR, et al. Normativa sobre Cirugía del Sistema Nervioso Simpático Torácico. Arch Bronchoneumol 2011; 47:94–102.

12. Ray WZ, Mackinnon SE. Management of nerve gaps: autografts, allografts, nerve transfers, and end-to-side neurorrhaphy. Exp Neurol 2010;223: 77–85.

13. Grinsell D, Keating CP. Peripheral nerve reconstruction after injury: a review of clinical and experimental therapies. Biomed Res Int 2014;2014:698256.

14. Terzis J, Faibishoff B, Williams B. The nerve gap: suture under tension vs graft. Plast Reconstr Surg 1975;56:166–70.

15. Purves D, Thompson W, Yip W. Re-innervation of ganglia transplanted to the neck from different levels of the guinea-pig sympathetic chain. J Physiol 1981; 313:49–63.

16. Matsumoto I, Kaneko M, Oda M, et al. Repair of intra-thoracic autonomic nerves using chitosan tubes. Interact Cardiovasc Thorac Surg 2010;10: 498–501.

17. Latif MJ, Afthinos JN, Connery CP, et al. Robotic intercostal nerve graft for reversal of thoracic sympathectomy: a large animal feasibility model. Int J Med Robot 2008;4:258–62.

18. Connery CP. Poster presentation 9th International Symposium on Sympathetic Surgery. Odense (Denmark), June 17–19, 2011.

19. Telaranta T. Secondary sympathetic chain reconstruction after endoscopic thoracic sympathicotomy. Eur J Surg 1998;(Suppl 580):17–8.

20. Telaranta T. Presentation 7th International Symposium on Sympathetic Surgery. Vienna (Austria), May 4–6, 2005.

21. Rantanen T, Telaranta T. Long-Term effect of endoscopic sympathetic nerve reconstruction for side effects after endoscopic sympathectomy. Thorac Cardiovasc Surg 2016. [Epub ahead of print].

22. Haam SJ, Seung YP, Paik HC, et al. Sympathetic nerve reconstruction for compensatory hyperhidrosis after sympathetic surgery for primary hyperhidrosis. J Korean Med Sci 2010;25:597–601.

23. Wong RHL, Ng CSH, Wong JKW, et al. Needlescopic video-assisted thoracic surgery for reversal of thoracic sympathectomy. Interact Cardiovasc Thorac Surg 2012;14:350–2.

24. Park HS, Hensman C, Leong J. Thoracic sympathetic nerve reconstruction for compensatory hyperhidrosis: the Melbourne technique. Ann Transl Med 2014;2(5):45.

25. Connery CP. Presentation 9th International Symposium on Sympathetic Surgery. Odense (Denmark), June 17–19, 2011.

26. Westphal FL, Milanez de Campos JR, Ribas M, et al. Skin depigmentation: could it be a complication caused by thoracic sympathectomy? Ann Thorac Surg 2009;88:e42–3.

27. Finlay AY, Khan GK. Dermatology life quality index (DLQI): a simple practical measure for routine clinical use. Clin Exp Dermatol 1994;19:210–6.

28. Brazier JE, Harper R, Jones NMB, et al. Validating the SF-36 health survey questionnaire: new outcome measure for primary care. BMJ 1992;305:160–4.

29. Cerfolio RJ, Bryant AS. Robotic-assisted pulmonary resection-right upper lobectomy. Ann Cardiothorac Surg 2012;1(1):77–85.

30. Connery CP. Presentation 11th International Symposium on Sympathetic Surgery. Santiago (Chile), October 15–16, 2015.

# Quality of Life Changes Following Surgery for Hyperhidrosis

José Ribas Milanez de Campos, MD, PhD[a,1],
Hugo Veiga Sampaio da Fonseca, MD[a,*],
Nelson Wolosker, MD, PhD[b,c]

## KEYWORDS

- Hyperhidrosis • Sympathectomy • Quality of life • Questioner in quality of life
- Compensatory hyperhidrosis

## KEY POINTS

- The best way to evaluate the impact of primary hyperhidrosis (PH) on quality of life (QL) is through specific questionnaires, avoiding generic models that do not appropriately evaluate individuals.
- A specific QL questionnaire for PH should comprise 4 domains: functional, social, interpersonal, and emotional.
- QL improves significantly in the short term after sympathectomy. In the longer term, a sustained and stable improvement is seen, although there is a small decline in the numbers; after 5 and even at 10 years of follow-up it shows virtually the same numerical distribution.
- Compensatory hyperhidrosis is a major side effect and the main aggravating factor in postoperative QL, requiring attention to its management and prevention.

## INTRODUCTION

Quality of life (QL) has various definitions and characteristics. It considers factors such as health, education, and physical, mental, and emotional well-being, among a number of other factors. QL includes human concerns and all that surrounds us: family, friends, and work. Additionally, QL is a subjective perception about one's position toward life, social and cultural context, values and expectations, standards and concerns. It is, therefore, too broad in scope, summing up conditions provided to each individual to live as intended.

According to the World Health Organization's (WHO) definition, from 1946, health is a state of complete physical, mental, and social well-being and not merely the absence of disease or infirmity.[1,2] As a result, an individual, even without presenting with any organic disturbance, needs to have QL to be considered healthy. Based on this assumption, the measurement of health cannot be bound by the absence of disease, but also should consider various wellness scales, as well as everyday problems and the social impact of health in daily life.

Disclosure Statement: The authors have nothing to disclose.
[a] Thoracic Surgery Division, Heart Institute/Clinics Hospital from University of São Paulo Medical School, 44 Dr. Enéas de Carvalho Aguiar Av., São Paulo 05403-000, São Paulo, Brazil; [b] Vascular Surgery Division, Albert Einstein Israelite Hospital, 627/701 Albert Einstein Avenue, Block A1, Room 423, Morumbi, São Paulo 05652-900, São Paulo, Brazil; [c] Vascular and Endovascular Division, Clinics Hospital from University of São Paulo Medical School, 225 Dr Ovídio Pires Campos St, Ambulatory Building, 6th floor, Unit 7B, São Paulo 05403-010, São Paulo, Brazil
[1] Present address: 44 Dr. Enéas de Carvalho Aguiar Av., Block 2, 2nd Floor, Room 9, São Paulo, São Paulo 05403-000, Brazil.
* Corresponding author. 103 José Paraíso St., Unit 902, Boa Viagem, Recife, Pernambuco 51030-390, Brazil.
E-mail address: veigasampaio@hotmail.com

1547-4127/16/© 2016 Elsevier Inc. All rights reserved.

This concern led to the search for a set of indicators that would track and represent the relationship between QL and health. More recently, a WHO study group developed a tool to assess QL in an international, cross-cultural perspective, consisting of 100 questions in the categories of physical, psychological, level of independence, social relationships, environment, and spiritual aspects (religion and personal beliefs). This instrument was named World Health Organization Quality of Life (WHOQOL-100).[1] Subsequently, to create a shorter and simpler instrument with faster time to completion, while maintaining satisfactory psychometric characteristics, a shorter questionnaire was created (WHOQOL-BREF). It contains 26 questions on physical, psychological, social relationships, and interaction with the environment.[3–8] These tools are generic, as they are not designed to evaluate topics typically affected by a specific health problem. However, there are other QL-related indicators to consider the impact of more specific conditions or diseases from different physical states, such as postoperative state and primary hyperhidrosis (PH).

## QUALITY OF LIFE AND HYPERHIDROSIS

Currently, QL has become an important factor to evaluate results in medicine. This psychosocial aspect is fundamental to help better manage patients, and can be more easily performed in serious illness. In cases of chronic and/or recurrent diseases with complex etiologies, including those with functional, emotional, social, psychological, and professional impact, this assessment must be performed with questionnaires. Most of these questionnaires are yet to be translated into Portuguese. At first sight, it seems clear that PH is one cause of subjective distress to patients, forcing them to live in a world in which sweating is considered unaesthetic and antisocial, especially for those who sweat much more than their physiologic needs.

In patients with severe palmar PH (dripping fingers), manipulating papers and other similar materials becomes virtually impossible. This condition is perceptible not only to the patient, but also to those around him or her, and can cause anxiety, suffering, and isolation. It can also be considered disabling and dangerous for certain professions. For example, policemen need to use weapons and electricians need to handle electrical or electronic materials. In addition, this condition can cause devastating consequences, not only in work but also in social activities, deteriorating QL.

Axillary PH is also considered a self-limiting disorder that leads individuals to social and psychological debilitation, interfering in affective aspect, and often causing isolation and depression. Bechara and colleagues[9] evaluated 51 patients with axillary PH. After 9 months of treatment, outcomes were evaluated, including a QL questionnaire. They concluded that surgical therapy could reverse almost 80% of disabilities caused by excessive axillary PH. The use of oxybutynin also offers satisfactory results.[10,11]

Craniofacial PH, with or without blushing, is a social and professionally embarrassing manifestation, as it gives an idea of weakness. When associated with social phobia or any other anxiety disorder, it is easier to recognize, increasing and aggravating psychiatric disorders.[12] Therefore, it is also considered a disorder that causes a steep decrease in QL.

Currently, video-assisted thoracic sympathectomy (VTS) is considered the safest and most effective treatment of PH, even in children and adolescents. Some studies treat patients even at 5 years of age.[13] Unlike other surgical procedures, which interfere directly in the target organ or diseased tissue, sympathetic denervation acts at a distance. This denervation stops the excessive stimulus that is responsible for sweating in the affected extremities. Current trends indicate VTS in children older than 7 years and before puberty due to exuberant symptoms. These symptoms can cause major social disturbance. Surgery is able to restore stable psychosocial development.

## QUALITY OF LIFE EVALUATION IN HYPERHIDROSIS

Several studies apply adapted questionnaires that associate QL and sympathectomy in the context of hyperhidrosis.[14–17] Such questionnaires include Medical Outcomes Study Short Form 36 (SF-36), Spielberger State Trait Anxiety Inventory (STAI), Zung Self-Rating Depression Scale (SDS), and the Dermatology Life Quality Index (DLQI). However, despite the easy applicability and relatively good validation through clinical studies, adapted questionnaires are limited in chronic diseases, such as PH, given its complexity and specificity. Even so, benefits of VTS to improve QL in these patients, especially in emotional and social aspects, are unquestionable.

As a result, we believe that a specific questionnaire is required to accurately assess QL in patients with PH. Amir and colleagues[18] described the early stages of preparing a specific health questionnaire to assess the impact of PH in QL of patients. We developed the first questionnaire specifically designed to assess QL in patients with PH who underwent VTS. There is no evidence that PH is a purely psychiatric disorder, admitting that psychological disorders, when present, are consequences of the constraints they experience from excessive sweating since early childhood.

Juniper and colleagues[19] wrote how to develop and validate new QL assessment tools related to health problems. Amir and colleagues[18] started the foundation for a specific PH questionnaire, as follows: interview PH candidates for surgery, from 15 to 35 years old, with different backgrounds and from diverse social classes. Two psychology student interviewers, focused to notice how PH could limit the patient's life, conducted this approach.

Patients were then encouraged to include all the situations they considered relevant in their social life, work, interpersonal, leisure, and any other activities in which they felt affected by the disorder. The interviewers, in the presence of a psychologist, psychiatrist, and the surgeon who selected the surgery group, reanalyzed all interviews. Four domains or functions had been identified as the most important: functional, social, interpersonal or relationships, and emotional. Emotion was divided into 2 areas: "self-emotional," the assessment of how PH impacts on himself or herself; and "other-emotional," evaluation of the patient's feeling about what others think about his or her problem. These areas were further defined by taking into consideration the various situations in which PH decisively interfered in the QL of the patient.

The major limitation of the study by Amir and colleagues,[18] recognized by the authors, was the selection bias. Because the populations studied were those already included in the official surgical line, only the most affected patients would be on this list. QL in patients with milder complaints may not be sharply affected.

## SPECIFIC QUALITY OF LIFE QUESTIONNAIRE FOR HYPERHIDROSIS: OUR EXPERIENCE

Based on previous work, we proposed our questionnaire, which was divided into 4 domains: functional-social, personal in relation to the partner, self-emotional and with others, and special conditions found to be important.

The first QL questionnaire assessment was performed before the patient's initial consultation. After, each patient received a handbook with information about PH, and the different options of clinical and surgical treatment. Additional information included expected results, complications, and problems that might occur postoperatively. After the consultation, examination, and election for surgical treatment, the patient was operated on. During the first 30 days after surgery, each patient answered the second part of the questionnaire. After a minimum period of 5 years, the patient was contacted by phone by a nurse, an independent observer, without access to the detailed medical records or the minutiae of the operation that had been held, and administered the late postoperative period questionnaire.

Analysis of questionnaire responses demonstrated that, in the preoperative period, 87.6% of patients rated QL as "bad" or "very bad". Thirty days later 96% classified QL as "better" or "little better," even after this short follow-up time.

Amir and colleagues[18] also found 3 interesting facts that were studied in our population. The first refers to the patient's gender: women initially showed a lower value in the QL questionnaire for most domains assessed when compared with men, except the emotional factor. This finding can perhaps be explained by women being faster to seek help and having easier emotional expression. In particular, men tend to behave as more tolerant of discomfort, especially with disorders with strong aesthetic connotation. In our population, there was no significant association between the answers related to QL and sex in both periods studied. Total distribution was very coincident, with similar variation in both men and women.

The second observation is related to the duration of symptoms: patients with PH since childhood showed lower QL than those in which the autonomic dysfunction arose after puberty, adolescence, or adulthood. The earlier the exposure of children to embarrassing social situations due to excessive sweating, the less social interaction experience, limiting social skill knowledge necessary to face problems. Corroborating this view, it is considered that for patients with PH, it is increasingly difficult to live or to get used to "embarrassing situations." Thus, the longer time with the disorder, the greater the loss of QL. In our sample, we found this trend because the responses to the QL questionnaire matched by age showed the most positive responses; that is, QL improvement tends to be more frequent in patients younger than 18 years. After 30 days, this difference was not significant; however, after 5 years, this difference was considered significant.

The third relevant observation is that the subjective distress is strongly related to the loss or damage suffered, particularly in the functional-social domain. This discomfort, even isolated, could result in an indication for a more aggressive and definitive treatment. Amir and colleagues[18] insist that surgeons in this field should take this fact into consideration when indicating surgery, and also when measuring intervention impact. To assess this outcome, the simplest way would be to ask patients to choose 3 domains in order of their preference. In each case, an idea of which domain had the biggest improvement on QL would be elucidated.

Among the chosen fields, we found that the most affected was the "functional-social," that is the one that relates to practical matters of everyday life. This observation was made in both early and late follow-up.[20] Moreover, this domain was one of the most chosen as first and second options, and even as a third. Thus, this questionnaire shows how PH negatively affects almost all routine activities. Other domains were also significantly changed, such as "personal," because patients felt much more confident in their personal relationships and places around them, soon after surgery. An important finding to notice is that the "emotional" domain was the second most chosen, indicating that the patients were extremely pleased to no longer justify their symptoms or face rejection from others.

A proposed QL questionnaire can be found in the supplementary section.

## RESULTS IN POSTOPERATIVE QUALITY OF LIFE

It is important to compare variations of QL, and its various aspects, to evaluate efficacy of PH treatment at different follow-up periods. The experiment described later in this article was based on analysis of QL questionnaires proposed by the expert consensus of the Society of Thoracic Surgeons published in the Annals of Surgery in 2011 for surgical treatment of PH.[21]

| Table 1 Surgical technique for hyperhidrosis | |
|---|---|
| Surgical Technique | Thoracic Ganglia |
| Palmar-plantar | T2 |
| Palmar-axillary-plantar | T2–T3 |
| Pure axillary | T3–T4 |
| Facial | T2 |

The main article,[20] which presents the questionnaire proposed in this article, received 107 citations in Web of Science and 134 citations in Scopus. The full version of this questionnaire is available at the end of this article.

### 30 Days of Follow-up

Between 1995 and 2002, 403 patients (62% women and 38% men) were submitted to VTS at Clinics Hospital from São Paulo University Medical School and were followed regarding QL changes, using the proposed questionnaire. Surgical resection levels or cauterization of the sympathetic chains were selected accordingly to clinical complaint (**Table 1**).

A total of 217 patients (57%) complained of plantar and palmar hyperhidrosis; 95 patients (25%) of palmar, axillary, and plantar hyperhidrosis; 60 patients (15.7%) only axillary PH; and 25 patients (6.5%) of facial PH.

The following represent (**Fig. 1**) patient responses for QL before and 30 days after surgery. Responses were divided as follows: "Better" in "MUCH BETTER" and "LITTLE BETTER"; "WORSE" in "LITTLE WORSE" and "MUCH WORSE."

From patients who considered QL as "GOOD" before surgery, 66.7% reported to be "MUCH BETTER" or "LITTLE BETTER." From patients who considered their QL as "BAD" before surgery,

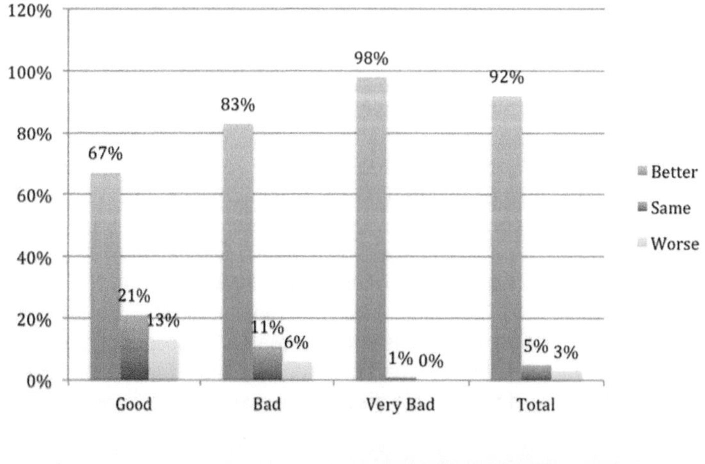

Fig. 1. QL improvement 30 days after surgery compared with preoperative initial status.

83.1% changed their answer to "MUCH BETTER" or "LITTLE BETTER." From those who classified QL as "VERY BAD," 98.3% reported to be "MUCH BETTER" or "LITTLE BETTER." From the total sample, 92% considered QL as at least "LITTLE BETTER" or "MUCH BETTER" after surgery. The worse the patient rated QL before surgery, the greater the patient felt the improvement.

## 5 Years of Follow-up

Below are QL before VTS and 5 years after the procedure (**Fig. 2**). From patients who considered QL as "GOOD" before surgery, 77% reported to be "MUCH BETTER" or "LITTLE BETTER." From patients who considered their QL as "BAD" before surgery, 84% changed their response to "MUCH BETTER" or "LITTLE BETTER." From those who classified QL as "VERY BAD," 93% reported to be "MUCH BETTER" or "LITTLE BETTER." From the total, 89% considered the QL as at least "LITTLE BETTER" or "MUCH BETTER" after 5 years of surgery. The worse the patient rated QL before surgery, the greater the patient felt the improvement.

Analysis in all patients between responses after 30 days and after 5 years of surgery showed statistically significant difference between distributions of answers in both periods (**Table 2**).

Thirty days after surgery, 75.5% of patients considered their QL as "much better." Five years later, this percentage decreased to 56.7%. However, 69.2% of patients maintained their opinions in both periods, 30.8% considered QL as "worse" than before, and 10.4% expressed as "better." This result ($P<.001$) is highly significant, indicating that there are differences between the 2 periods when comparing the responses.

It is necessary to point out that the differences found are between the categories "MUCH BETTER" and "LITTLE BETTER." The frequency of "MUCH BETTER" decreased, while "LITTLE BETTER" increased from one period to another. We highlight that if only 2 categories of answers ("BETTER" and "SAME or WORSE") are considered, 92% of answers were "BETTER" at 30 days and 90.6% within 5 years. These numbers show that despite the difference in the 2 periods, it is very important to notice the immediate change to "BETTER" and the maintenance of this improvement in QL after 5 years of VTS.

## 10 Years of Follow-up

Currently, we have more than 500 patients under follow-up who underwent surgery in the same period in which the study of 5 years was conducted. Now, after 10 years of follow-up, the results remain similar for improvement in QL. In a total of 513 patients studied, the category MUCH BETTER has 55.9% of the patients, 34.8% of "LITTLE BETTER," "SAME" with 3.2%, "LITTLE WORSE" of approximately 3% and "MUCH WORSE" with 3.1%. If continued with the same numbers, then the patients experience 90.7% of better QL after 10 years of thoracic sympathectomy. This confirms the initial improvement, and can be considered stable for patients in whom it has been achieved. On the other hand, we observe a slight change in results: "SAME" fell from 6.8% to 3.2%; "LITTLE WORSE" from 1.1%, rose to 3.0%; "MUCH WORSE" also rose from 1.4% to 3.1%. These results are currently under interpretation to understand a difference found in gender. So far, this difference is linked to a gradual increase in body mass index (BMI) after 10 years, rather than any other studied factor (**Fig. 3**).

## IMPACT OF COMPENSATORY HYPERHIDROSIS IN QUALITY OF LIFE AFTER SURGERY

Compensatory hyperhidrosis (CH) may occur with any level of sympathectomy and patients report

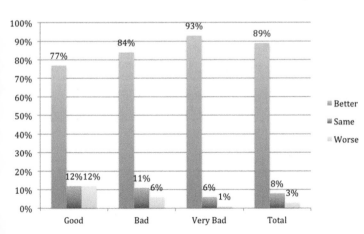

Fig. 2. QL improvement 5 years after surgery compared with preoperative initial status.

**Table 2**
**McNemar test to compare both moments (after 30 days and 5 years of surgery) relative to the QL answers**

| Category | Total (30 d), n (%) | Total (5 y), n (%) |
|---|---|---|
| Much better | 75.5 | 56.7 |
| Little better | 16.5 | 33.9 |
| Same | 5.1 | 6.8 |
| Little worse | 1.7 | 1.1 |
| Much worse | 1.1 | 1.4 |

McNemar test: P<.001.

different symptom intensities. When it is of low magnitude (almost all patients submitted VTS will develop it), it has no effects on the QL questionnaire. It is necessary to be intense and interfere in daily activities to counteract the good results related to the main complaint. In these cases, patients will regret the VTS,[22] as we found in our study, in which most patients who reported no satisfaction with surgical treatment mentioned CH as the cause.

Regarding the development of CH, we found the following: 15 (3.7%) did not report any occurrence of CH; 57 (14.1%) reported it as mild; 174 (43.2%) as moderate; 150 (37.2%) as intense; and only 7 (1.7%) of them were unhappy and reported regretting undergoing the surgical procedure. After 10 years of follow-up, these numbers are slightly higher, as suggested in previous paragraphs, and so far are being considered to be the result of an increase in BMI.

Abundant compensatory sweating can be a cause of regret related to surgery, and consequently a reduction in QL rates. In some cases, despite this manifestation, many of our patients

revealed high satisfaction with VTS. These data reflect not only our personal experience, but also those reported by several international centers.[22,23] There is no clinical or laboratory test that allows safe prediction of CH intensity. Hence, there is a need to warn all patients with PH about these unpleasant effects, which are difficult to control with currently available therapies. We emphasize that, even after VTS, the structure of sweat glands remains intact. The interruption of sympathetic preganglionic fibers does not prevent sweat secretion, either by stimulation of postganglionic fibers or by local administration of cholinergic agents.

In the past few years, there is a tendency among surgeons to limit the number of sympathetic ganglia removed, and, perhaps most important step, to avoid greater resections, including the second ganglion (G2). In our clinic, from the beginning, we established the G2 approach for craniofacial PH. For palmar PH, we initially used to approach G2 and G3 nodes. Over the past years, we focused only in the G3. For axillary PH, we initially worked on G3 and G4, but soon after we started to intervene only on G4.

CH is really an important issue and has negative impact on patient QL. Fujita and colleagues[24] investigated whether increased palmar temperature and blood flow observed during surgery could be a predictive factor for the development of CH in the postoperative period. Twenty-seven patients were consecutively monitored, finding a significant correlation between development of CH and an increase of palmar temperature and blood flow to the extremities. With a higher increase in both variables, there is a greater chance for patients to present with CH.

Indeed, CH may occur after section at any level of the sympathetic chain, despite the number of nodes resected. Our personal observation over

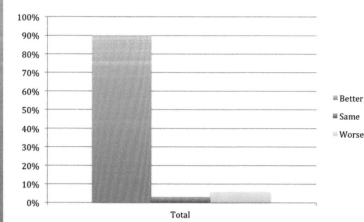

**Fig. 3.** QL improvement 10 years after surgery comparing with preoperative initial status, without distinguishing the preoperative status QL.

12 years is that the higher the level of the sectioned chain, for example, the G2 level, the greater the hand temperature during surgery, secondary to increased blood flow in the denervated area. This occurrence can be noticed only during VTS. As a result, there may be more severe CH. When VTS is performed in lower levels, such as G3 or G4, we cannot always notice an increase in temperature of the hand during surgery.

## SUMMARY

- When PH directly affects an individual's QL, it should be addressed not only as a medical problem, but also as a mental, psychological, professional, and social disorder.
- The best way to evaluate the impact of PH on QL is through specific questionnaires, avoiding generic models that do not appropriately evaluate individuals.
- VTS is the most effective therapy for short-term and long-term control of symptoms, with major impact on QL.
- A specific QL questionnaire for PH should comprise 4 domains: functional, social, interpersonal, and emotional.
- Generally women have their quality of life more affected than men, except in the emotional field due to their cultural characteristic to seek professional help faster.
- Hyperhidrosis in childhood is accompanied with negative impact on long-term QL, when compared with those whose symptoms started in adolescence or early adulthood.
- The higher the impact on QL, the greater the demand and patient's perseverance to pursue a more aggressive and definitive treatment.
- Among the chosen domains, we found that the most mentioned was the "functional-social"; that is, the one that relates to daily life.
- The QL questionnaire proposed in this article has wide acceptance in the literature and is recommended by Consensus of the Society of Thoracic Surgeons; we consider it easy to understand by patients and it has shown effective results when analyzing different periods of follow-up.
- QL improves significantly in the short term after sympathectomy. In the longer term, a sustained and stable improvement is seen, although there is a small decline in the numbers; after 5 and even at 10 years of follow-up it shows virtually the same numerical distribution.
- CH is a major side effect and the main aggravating factor in postoperative QL, requiring attention to its management and prevention.

- Prevention of CH involves a good characterization of the patient's complaints and its impact on QL so as to select the correct level for interruption of the sympathetic chain.

## REFERENCES

1. World Health Organization. Preamble to the Constitution of the World Health Organization as adopted by the International Health Conference [Internet]. Official Records of the World Health Organization. 1946. p. 100. Available at: http://www.who.int/governance/eb/who_constitution_en.pdf. Accessed July 31, 2016.
2. Group TW. Development of the World Health Organization WHOQOL-BREF quality of life assessment. The WHOQOL Group. Psychol Med 1998;28(3):551–8.
3. The World Health Organization Quality of Life Assessment (WHOQOL): development and general psychometric properties. Soc Sci Med 1998;46(12):1569–85.
4. De Campos JRM, Kauffman P, Werebe EC, et al. Questionário de qualidade de vida em pacientes com hiperidrose primária. J Pneumol 2003;29:178–81.
5. Elia S, Guggino G, Mineo D, et al. Awake one stage bilateral thoracoscopic sympathectomy for palmar hyperhidrosis: a safe outpatient procedure. Eur J Cardiothorac Surg 2005;28(2):312–7 [discussion: 317].
6. Kauffman P, Milanez JRC, Jatene FB. Simpatectomia cervicotorácica por videotoracoscopia: experiência inicial. Rev Col Bras Cir 1998;25:235–9.
7. Tu YR, Li X, Lin M, et al. Epidemiological survey of primary palmar hyperhidrosis in adolescent in Fuzhou of People's Republic of China. Eur J Cardiothorac Surg 2007;31(4):737–9.
8. Strutton DR, Kowalski JW, Glaser DA, et al. US prevalence of hyperhidrosis and impact on individuals with axillary hyperhidrosis: results from a national survey. J Am Acad Dermatol 2004;51(2):241–8.
9. Bechara FG, Gambichler T, Bader A, et al. Assessment of quality of life in patients with primary axillary hyperhidrosis before and after suction-curettage. J Am Acad Dermatol 2007;57(2):207–12.
10. Wolosker N, de Campos JR, Kauffman P, et al. An alternative to treat palmar hyperhidrosis: use of oxybutynin. Clin Auton Res 2011;21(6):389–93.
11. Wolosker N, Campos JR, Kauffman P, et al. The use of oxybutynin for treating facial hyperhidrosis. An Bras Dermatol 2011;86(3):451–6.
12. Sciuchetti JF, Ballabio D, Corti F, et al. Endoscopic thoracic sympathectomy by clamping in the treatment of social phobia: the Monza experience. Minerva Chir 2006;61(5):417–20.
13. Lin TS. Transthoracic endoscopic sympathectomy for palmar hyperhidrosis in children and adolescents: analysis of 350 cases. J Laparoendosc Adv Surg Tech A 1999;9(4):331–4.

14. Kumagai K, Kawase H, Kawanishi M. Health-related quality of life after thoracoscopic sympathectomy for palmar hyperhidrosis. Ann Thorac Surg 2005;80(2): 461–6.

15. Swan MC, Paes T. Quality of life evaluation following endoscopic transthoracic sympathectomy for upper limb and facial hyperhydrosis. Ann Chir Gynaecol 2001;90(3):157–9.

16. Lau WT, Lee JD, Dang CR, et al. Improvement in quality of life after bilateral transthoracic endoscopic sympathectomy for palmar hyperhydrosis. Hawaii Med J 2001;60(5):126, 137.

17. Fredman B, Zohar E, Shachor D, et al. Video-assisted transthoracic sympathectomy in the treatment of primary hyperhidrosis: friend or foe? Surg Laparosc Endosc Percutan Tech 2000;10(4):226–9.

18. Amir M, Arish A, Weinstein Y, et al. Impairment in quality of life among patients seeking surgery for hyperhidrosis (excessive sweating): preliminary results. Isr J Psychiatry Relat Sci 2000;37(1):25–31.

19. Juniper EF, Guyatt GH, Streiner DL, et al. Clinical impact versus factor analysis for quality of life questionnaire construction. J Clin Epidemiol 1997;50(3): 233–8.

20. de Campos JRM, Kauffman P, Werebe Ede C, et al. Quality of life, before and after thoracic sympathectomy: report on 378 operated patients. Ann Thorac Surg 2003;76(3):886–91.

21. Cerfolio RJ, De Campos JRM, Bryant AS, et al. The Society of Thoracic Surgeons expert consensus for the surgical treatment of hyperhidrosis. Ann Thorac Surg 2011;91(5):1642–8.

22. Libson S, Kirshtein B, Mizrahi S, et al. Evaluation of compensatory sweating after bilateral thoracoscopic sympathectomy for palmar hyperhidrosis. Surg Laparosc Endosc Percutan Tech 2007;17(6):511–3.

23. Ribas Milanez de Campos J, Kauffman P, Wolosker N, et al. Axillary hyperhidrosis: T3/T4 versus T4 thoracic sympathectomy in a series of 276 cases. J Laparoendosc Adv Surg Tech A 2006;16(6):598–603.

24. Fujita T, Mano M, Nishi H, et al. Intraoperative prediction of compensatory sweating for thoracic sympathectomy. Jpn J Thorac Cardiovasc Surg 2005; 53(9):481–5.

## APPENDIX 1: QUALITY OF LIFE FULL QUESTIONNAIRE

This questionnaire must be completed fully before and after surgery at different time points (Appendix 1). As the authors emphasize, the suggestion is to use the questionnaire after 30 days, 5 years, and 10 years of intervention.

The first portion (see **Tables 1** and **2**) is the direct question to the patient, who will answer about QL globally before surgery, and how it has changed with the VTS, for better or for worse. This answer is given in 5 levels that are equivalent for comparison purposes.

The second part supports a detailed analysis of 4 different domains, made in collaboration with Amir and colleagues.[18] The system consists of a scale ranging between 20 and 100 points in the analyzed periods. Each of these domains or group of functions contains 5 levels based on tables that result in only one answer.

Preoperatively, when the sum of the points was greater than 84, QL was classified as "VERY BAD"; 84-69, "BAD"; 68-53, "GOOD"; 52-36, "VERY GOOD"; and 20-35, as "EXCELLENT." In the postoperative analysis we have used the periods of 30 days, 5 years, and 10 years. When the sum was greater than 84 points, QL was classified as "MUCH WORSE"; 84-69, "LITTLE WORSE"; of 68 to 53, "SAME"; 52-36, "LITTLE BETTER"; and 20-35, as "MUCH BETTER."

The difference between preoperative and the 2 other evaluations obtained in the postoperative period was named as "the effect of early and late surgical treatment in QL of patients."

### HEALTH RELATED QUESTIONNAIRE – HYPERHIDROSIS

NAME: ............................................................DATE......./......./.......
Date of the Surgical Procedure: .........../.........../...........

This study is RESTRICTED TO QUESTIONS CONCERNING YOUR WELL-BEING AND LIFE QUALITY, BEFORE AND AFTER SURGERY FOR CORRECTION OF HYPERHIDROSIS AND OR FACIAL BLUSHING/SWETTING. This information is important because we want to know how you feel and how well you are able to conduct your daily activities. Please answer each question marking only the answer as indicated. If you are in doubt about the answer, reread the question and try to answer to the best of your ability.

**TABLE 01.**    **Generally speaking, how would you rate your life quality BEFORE SURGERY?**

| | |
|---|---|
| Excellent | 1 |
| Very good | 2 |
| Good | 3 |
| Poor/Inferior | 4 |
| Very poor/Inferior | 5 |

**TABLE 02.**    **Compared to the period before surgery how would you rate your life quality AT LEAST 30 DAYS AFTER SURGERY?**

| | |
|---|---|
| Much better | 1 |
| Slightly better | 2 |
| The same | 3 |
| Slightly worse | 4 |
| Much worse | 5 |

**ATTENTION:** STARTING FROM THE NEXT QUESTION, PLEASE ALWAYS USE THE SCALE OF VALUES USED IN THE TWO TABLES ABOVE, SELECTING ONLY ONE CHOICE FOR EACH ANSWER. THIS QUESTIONNAIRE IS CONFIDENTIAL AND WILL BE UTILIZED ONLY FOR STUDY PURPOSES.

**1)    FUNCTIONAL / SOCIAL DOMAIN, with relation to the following items, how would you rate your quality of life:**

| | Before surgery: | After surgery: |
|---|---|---|
| Writing: | 1 2 3 4 5 | 1 2 3 4 5 |
| Doing manual work: | 1 2 3 4 5 | 1 2 3 4 5 |
| Doing recreation: | 1 2 3 4 5 | 1 2 3 4 5 |
| Doing sports: | 1 2 3 4 5 | 1 2 3 4 5 |
| Shaking hands: | 1 2 3 4 5 | 1 2 3 4 5 |
| Being with friends (public places): | 1 2 3 4 5 | 1 2 3 4 5 |
| Grasping objects: | 1 2 3 4 5 | 1 2 3 4 5 |
| Social dancing: | 1 2 3 4 5 | 1 2 3 4 5 |

**2)    PERSONAL DOMAIN, with your partner / spouse. How would you rate your quality of life:**

| | Before surgery: | After surgery: |
|---|---|---|
| Holding hands: | 1 2 3 4 5 | 1 2 3 4 5 |
| Intimate touching: | 1 2 3 4 5 | 1 2 3 4 5 |
| Intimate affairs: | 1 2 3 4 5 | 1 2 3 4 5 |

**3)    EMOTIONAL-SELF or OTHERS; how would you rate the fact that after sweating/blushing excessively:**

| | Before surgery: | After surgery: |
|---|---|---|
| I always justified myself: | 1 2 3 4 5 | 1 2 3 4 5 |
| People rejected you slightly: | 1 2 3 4 5 | 1 2 3 4 5 |

**4)    UNDER SPECIAL CIRCUMSTANCES – How would you rate your quality of life:**

| | Before surgery: | After surgery: |
|---|---|---|
| In a closed or hot environment: | 1 2 3 4 5 | 1 2 3 4 5 |
| When tense or worried: | 1 2 3 4 5 | 1 2 3 4 5 |
| Thinking about the problem: | 1 2 3 4 5 | 1 2 3 4 5 |
| Before an examination/meeting/speaking in public: | 1 2 3 4 5 | 1 2 3 4 5 |
| Wearing sandals /walking barefoot: | 1 2 3 4 5 | 1 2 3 4 5 |
| Wearing colored clothing: | 1 2 3 4 5 | 1 2 3 4 5 |
| Having problems at school / work: | 1 2 3 4 5 | 1 2 3 4 5 |

# Management of Compensatory Sweating After Sympathetic Surgery

Nelson Wolosker, MD, PhD[a,b],
José Ribas Milanez de Campos, MD, PhD[c,d],
Juliana Maria Fukuda, MD[a,*]

## KEYWORDS

- Hyperhidrosis • Sweating • Sympathectomy • Sympathetic nervous system
- Cholinergic antagonists

## KEY POINTS

- Compensatory hyperhidrosis consists of an increase in the severity of sweating much more than necessary to regulate body temperature in locations that were previously normal.
- Compensatory hyperhidrosis is the most common and feared side effect of thoracic sympathectomy, because patients with severe forms have their quality of life greatly impaired.
- It is currently postulated that the occurrence of compensatory hyperhidrosis is a reflex mechanism, mediated by the hypothalamus.
- The most well-known factors associated with compensatory hyperhidrosis are extension of manipulation of the sympathetic chain, level of sympathetic denervation, and body mass index.
- Therapeutic options include topical agents, botulinum toxin, systemic anticholinergics, clip removal, and sympathetic chain reconstruction.

## INTRODUCTION

Sympathectomies have been performed for many decades for the treatment of hyperhidrosis (HH). Technical developments, like the advent of video-assisted operations in the 1990s, have brought safety and positive results to the procedure, leading to an overwhelming increase in the number of video-assisted thoracoscopic sympathectomies (VATS) in recent years.[1,2] In contrast, the postoperative phenomenon of compensatory HH (CH) has been observed more frequently, with an incidence ranging up to 98% in the literature.[3–10]

The wide variability in the incidence of CH may be attributable to heterogeneous patient populations, a variety of techniques of sympathetic denervation, or more important to a lack of objective methodology for defining CH.[11] CH was first described in 1935 by Adson and colleagues[12] and consists of an increase in the severity of sweating much more than necessary to regulate body temperature in locations that were previously normal.

---

The authors have nothing to disclose.
a Division of Vascular and Endovascular Surgery, Hospital Israelita Albert Einstein, Av. Albert Einstein, 627 – Bloco A1, 4° Andar, Sala 423 – Morumbi, São Paulo CEP 05652-000, Brazil; b Division of Vascular and Endovascular Surgery, Hospital das Clínicas da Faculdade de Medicina da Universidade de São Paulo, R. Dr. Enéas de Carvalho Aguiar, 255 – Instituto Central, 9° Andar, Sala 9117 – Cerqueira César, São Paulo CEP 05403-000, Brazil; c Division of Thoracic Surgery, Hospital Israelita Albert Einstein, Av. Albert Einstein, 627 – Bloco A1, 4° Andar, Sala 423 – Morumbi, São Paulo CEP 05652-000, Brazil; d Division of Thoracic Surgery, Hospital das Clínicas da Faculdade de Medicina da Universidade de São Paulo, R. Dr. Enéas de Carvalho Aguiar, 255 – Instituto Central, 9° Andar, Sala 9117 – Cerqueira César, São Paulo CEP 05403-000, Brazil
* Corresponding author.
E-mail address: ju_mfukuda@yahoo.com

1547-4127/16/© 2016 Elsevier Inc. All rights reserved.

thoracic.theclinics.com

CH occurs mainly in the abdomen, back, chest, and thighs, but may also be manifested on the feet, although the latter is infrequent. Most patients present with a combination of 2 or more areas.[13,14] CH is generally symmetric and usually occurs within 1 to 5 days after sympathectomy. It becomes more uncomfortable on hot days, in hot environments, during physical exercise, and when experiencing emotional stress and anxiety. It may diminish over time or the patient may learn to live with it.[15,16] CH is the most common and most feared side effect of thoracic sympathectomy.

In most cases, CH is tolerable and does not reach the point of social embarrassment or occupational disability. However, CH can be severely debilitating for some patients, leading them to regret the procedure in severe cases.[17] Patients with severe CH have their quality of life (QOL) greatly impaired, needing several changes of clothes during the day, and on very hot days, patients may avoid leaving home. CH is the Achilles' heel of sympathectomy, as many as 11.2% of patients expressed either dissatisfaction or regret about undergoing the procedure as a result of the occurrence of this troublesome consequence.[18]

## PATHOPHYSIOLOGY

The exact mechanism of the development of CH remains unknown. Shoenfeld and colleagues[19] suggested that the total amount of sweat produced did not vary after sympathectomy; however, the increase in perspiration in other parts of the body would represent a body's compensation for sympathetic denervation. Consequently, the term "CH" was adopted. Nevertheless, it is currently postulated that the occurrence of CH is a reflex mechanism, mediated by the hypothalamus after sympathetic surgery, and not a compensatory mechanism.[9,16,20]

Anatomically, the thermoregulatory sweat response is regulated by the hypothalamus, more precisely in the preoptic region. The sympathetic nerves originate in the intermediolateral horns of the spinal cord, between T1 and L2. Each sympathetic pathway is composed of preganglionic and postganglionic neurons. The nerve fibers to the sweat glands are postganglionic fibers. These fibers may go upward and downward in the sympathetic trunks before leaving and distributing to the sweat glands. Consequently, the distributions overlap and are not necessarily to the same part of the body from the same spinal segments.[21]

According to Chou and colleagues[22] changes in sweating patterns after sympathetic procedures may be attributable to a reflex response in the sweating center of the hypothalamus. Afferent negative feedback impulses initiated in the sweat glands stimulate sweating centers located in the hypothalamus, from where efferent positive feedback signals return to the target organs (eg, hands, soles, and armpits).

Sympathectomy at the T2 level causes a complete interruption of the negative feedback to the hypothalamus, contributing to the appearance of CH in peripheral areas owing to the magnified efferent signals originating from the hypothalamus, as well as the fact that the amplified sympathetic signals do not reach the sympathectomized areas. When performing sympathectomy at the T4 level, most of the afferent fibers are not damaged and the efferent stimuli are weaker; therefore, there are fewer cases of severe CH.

## CLASSIFICATION

To date, no consensus has been established concerning the classification of CH.[22] Although some authors count only cases in which massive overperspiration occurs, others consider even a slight increase in perspiration as CH.[23] Some authors believe that the increase in sweating in hot environments or during physical exercise is CH, whereas others state that this sweating is only a thermoregulatory response, thus being named compensatory sweating, leaving the term "CH" for more severe cases.[24]

The classification proposed by Gossot and colleagues[25] described 3 different intensity levels of CH (slight/mild, moderate/disturbing, and severe/disabling). Slight or mild CH was considered present when patients reported minor changes in the location and severity of their sweating, such as visible sweating during hot weather and when exercising, but without expressing significant concern. Moderate or disturbing CH was considered present when patients reported visible and embarrassing sweating or occasionally disabling situations caused by sweating. Severe or disabling CH was considered present when patients reported interference in their social and professional activities, such as the need for successive changes of clothes caused by sweating at the same intensity as their previous main site of HH, but at other primary locations.

Dumont and colleagues[26] defined 4 intensity levels of CH (low, moderate, severe, and very severe). Yazbek and colleagues[9] graded the severity of CH as severe or nonsevere. CH was considered to be severe if it was visible, embarrassing, and required more than 1 change of clothes during the day.

## PROPHYLAXIS

The ideal outcome of sympathectomy is that the patient can show adequate anhidrosis at the lowest quantity and severity of CH. Unfortunately, this optimal result is not achieved for all patients, which is why surgeons have been searching for risk factors and prophylactic strategies to prevent CH. To date, the most well-known factors associated with CH are extension of manipulation of the sympathetic chain, level of sympathetic denervation, and body mass index (BMI).

Several publications have reported the association between the severity of CH and the level, as well as the extension of sympathectomy.[8,20,22,27–29] It has been shown that upper levels of sympathectomy and more extensive manipulation of the sympathetic chain are directly related to more severe cases of CH. This is in compliance with the theory that CH results from the lack of the negative feedback to the hypothalamus after sympathectomy.

CH is more pronounced when patients are operated on at the T2 level, where there is an increasing convergence of afferent pathways to the hypothalamus. Some authors suggest that the preservation of the afferent pathway, which is responsible for the negative feedback to the hypothalamus, would be the fundamental factor to reduce CH rates in the postoperative period.[20,30] Hence, manipulation of a single ganglion should be performed for each site of HH, and intervention at lower ganglion levels (T4 for palmar and axillary HH) minimizes the chance of developing severe CH, leading to an improvement in QOL.

Munia and colleagues[29] reported reduced incidence of moderate or severe CH (34.3% for T3-T4 and 6.6% for T4; $P < .001$) and similar high efficacy when sympathectomy was performed at the T4 level for axillary HH, compared with the T3 to T4 level.

Liu and colleagues[30] published a study with patients with palmar HH, comparing 2 levels of sympathicotomy (T3 vs T4). The procedure was similarly effective for both groups, but the incidence of moderate/disturbing CH was lower (14.5% for T3 and 2.9% for T4; $P < .017$) for the patients operated on at the T4 level.

Li and colleagues[8] compared patients with palmar HH as a main complaint who underwent sympathectomy at the T3 level to those who were operated on at the T2 to T4 level showing that, despite the same high resolution rate for palmar HH, severe CH was lower (10% for T2-T4 and 3% for T3; $P < .05$) for the patients who received T3 denervation.

The relationship between sweating and BMI has been investigated before. It has been observed that individuals who are overweight or obese (BMI > 25.0 kg/m$^2$) present with more severe sweating than the general population, possibly as a result of reduced heat loss owing to thicker layers of fat in the subcutaneous tissue. Overweight and obese patients have a greater difficulty in maintaining normal body temperature and therefore produce excessive perspiration as a compensatory mechanism.[31] Another study showed that the greater the BMI for palmar and axillary HH, the greater the degree of CH after surgery.[7] For these reasons, there is a recommendation to operate only on patients classified as having a normal BMI to prevent severe cases of CH.

Currently, the best surgical method for sympathetic chain denervation, either cutting or clamping, remains controversial, although both methods have good results if the level of approach is correctly achieved. Differences in outcomes may be explained by a few reasons. The number of clips used to interrupt the sympathetic chain may vary across clamping procedures, affecting the effectiveness of treatment. Furthermore, the clamping method may have the potential loss of efficacy over time. In contrast, during cutting procedures, diathermic damage of collateral sympathetic fibers may cause a more pronounced denervation, aggravating CH.[32]

Some publications have reported a lower degree of sweating resolution, but a reduced incidence of CH, for the clamping technique,[32,33] whereas other studies have shown that not only the success rate, but also the rate of CH seemed to be the same for both methods.[34–36]

Reisfeld and colleagues[37] reported that the rate of severe CH was significantly lower in the clamping group than in the cutting groups (3% for clamping, and 6% and 8% for cutting; $P \leq .001$).

Children better tolerate the occurrence and severity of CH and their postoperative satisfaction rate is higher than that of adolescents and adults. Therefore, when indicated, VATS should be performed in children as early as possible.[38]

Some authors have used robotic surgery to reduce CH after VATS. Coveliers and colleagues[39] have shown that robotic thoracoscopic selective sympathectomy yields excellent relief of HH and low rates of CH (7.2%) and complications. Robotic surgical systems have the advantage of magnified high-definition 3-dimensional visualization and increased instrument maneuverability in a confined space, making it possible to perform division of the postganglionic sympathetic fibers. However, these robotic systems are expensive and thus accessibility is limited.

Because of the importance of CH, it is necessary to make all patients with HH aware of this risk before they choose sympathetic denervation over other available approaches. Although nearly all patients who are indicated for surgical treatment of HH have a poor QOL, this is a benign condition. Consequently, it is extremely important to explain to the patient, before surgery, the chance of side effects. Particularly, it is an obligation to emphasize that CH is a side effect that occurs in almost all cases, mostly in slight forms, but is permanent after surgery.[40]

## TREATMENT

Early diagnosis to enable early treatment is essential to deal with CH, aiming to prevent or reduce the incidence of psychological trauma and to improve QOL. The current treatment modalities for CH are summarized in **Box 1**. In addition to the orientation provided by the surgeon, it is highly recommended that a multidisciplinary team evaluate the patient.[3]

### Nonpharmacologic Treatment

Patients with CH should be instructed to maintain their BMI within the normal range (19.1–25.8 kg/m$^2$ for women and 20.7–26.4 kg/m$^2$ for men) because increases in BMI have a high correlation with greater sweating. Regular physical activity contributes to weight loss and a reduction in BMI.[7]

---

**Box 1**
**Treatment modalities**

*Nonpharmacologic*

Weight control

Regular physical activity

Nonthermogenic diet

*Pharmacologic*

Topical

    Aluminum chloride hexahydrate solutions

    Topical glycopyrrolate

Botulinum toxin

Systemic anticholinergics

    Oral glycopyrrolate

    Oxybutynin

*Surgical*

Clip removal

Sympathetic chain reconstruction

---

Certain foods, which are called thermogenic, have been reported to be sympathetic activators, stimulating an increase in body sweating. Examples of these foods, that should be avoided include chocolate, coffee, tea, pepper, cinnamon, ginger, milk and dairy products, and a high protein and carbohydrate diet. For this reason, the adoption of a nonthermogenic diet is considered an alternative to reduce CH. Patients with CH show improvement in sweating in cold environments with low humidity and good ventilation. The moderate climate of mountain towns can also be beneficial for patients.[3]

### Pharmacologic Treatment

#### Topical agents

Aluminum chloride hexahydrate solutions are available in 15% to 25% concentrations and can be used to treat large surface areas, with the main limitation being skin irritation. These products can be applied initially to affected areas once daily, at bedtime, and washed off in the morning, and increased as required to reduce symptoms.[3]

Another agent that can be administered is topical glycopyrrolate. It is an anticholinergic agent that does not cross the blood–brain barrier and has a slower penetration of tissue membranes than other drugs within its class, hence, producing fewer side effects. The main side effects when used topically are dry mouth, headache, sore throat, and mild skin dryness or irritation.[41] The use of topical treatment is an option; however, the effects are not permanent, thus offering unsatisfactory results.

#### Botulinum toxin

Botulinum toxin A is a neurotoxin produced by the anaerobic bacterium *Clostridium botulinum*. When used to treat HH, botulinum toxin is injected intradermally and acts to inhibit the release of acetylcholine at the neuromuscular junction and from sympathetic nerves that innervate eccrine sweat glands, which results in improvement in sweating.[42]

Contraindications to botulinum toxin therapy include skin infections and allergies to any of the ingredients, and neuromuscular disorders such as myasthenia gravis, pregnancy, lactation, and medications that may interfere with neuromuscular transmission.[43]

The major limitations of this technique are that the injections are painful and require local anesthesia, and the high cost of the drug inhibits its wider use for large areas of involvement, which are common in patients with CH. In addition, botulinum toxin has a temporary effect ranging from 4 to 17 months and it must be readministered periodically.[44]

Complications include headache, myalgia, itching, and the common cold for patients with axillary HH, and handgrip weakness and finger tingling and numbness for patients with palmar HH.[44–47] Patients should be referred to physicians specialized in the administration of botulinum toxin.

A case series with 17 patients reported the use of botulinum toxin A injection in the trunk, with complete resolution of CH within 5 days in 88.2% of the patients.[48] Other studies have shown good results in the management of CH, by reporting the use of botulinum toxin A injection in the chest, back, and abdomen,[49] as well as the use of endoscopic administration of botulinum toxin A to the sympathetic chain for CH in the trunk and legs.[50]

There is a controversy regarding the role of dilution volume, injection depth, type of skin, and amount of previous sweating, as well as application site in determining anhidrotic effects. New controlled studies with a greater number of patients are needed to draw solid conclusions. The results from the experiences described in these case reports and uncontrolled case series still need to be confirmed by controlled studies.

### Systemic anticholinergics

A systemic approach seems to be an adequate alternative, because CH may occur in large surface areas and usually occurs in more than 1 area simultaneously. Orally administered anticholinergic drugs have been used for at least the past 20 years, with considerably positive results in the treatment of HH.[51–54] They work by competitive inhibition of acetylcholine at muscarinic receptors near the eccrine sweat glands.

Contraindications include narrow angle glaucoma, myasthenia gravis, pyloric stenosis, and paralytic ileus. Common side effects of anticholinergic agents when given systemically include dry mouth, visual disturbance, urinary retention and urgency, flushing, constipation, tachycardia, and dizziness.[55]

Gong and colleagues[56] have studied the use of oral glycopyrrolate in 19 patients with CH, showing a significant improvement in QOL. During the 1-month follow-up, none of the patients stopped taking the medication, and the main side effect was dry mouth.

Teivelis and colleagues[57] reported the use of oxybutynin in 21 patients with CH. Oxybutynin was taken in progressively higher doses: starting at 2.5 mg once daily, then increased to twice daily after 1 week, and 5 mg twice daily at the third week. If necessary and tolerated, the total dose was increased to 20 mg/d. Five patients withdrew from the study for intolerability owing to anticholinergic side effects (mainly dry mouth) or lack of improvement in HH. All patients had significant improvement in sweating, with more than 70% reporting improved QOL.

An uncontrolled case series reported the use of botulinum toxin associated with oxybutynin for the treatment of CH, with a high positive impact on QOL. The trunk was the most common hyperhidrotic area of CH.[58] The current role of oral anticholinergic agents for the treatment of CH is not entirely clear, but seems to be a promising therapy. Further controlled studies with more patients and longer follow-up periods are required to validate these results.

### Surgical Treatment

It has been presented that clip removal and sympathetic chain reconstruction have a potential for reversibility.[59,60]

## SUMMARY

CH is the most frequent and is considered the most feared side effect of VATS. Technical developments as well as the proper selection of patients for surgery have been crucial in reducing the occurrence of severe forms of CH. Prophylactic measures include performing lower levels of sympathetic denervation and not indicating surgery for overweight and obese patients. The use of anticholinergic agents is the most effective pharmacologic treatment and botulinum toxin application is a therapeutic option to be considered in selected cases. Clip removal and sympathetic chain reconstruction are feasible alternatives, although their efficacy is not well-established.

## REFERENCES

1. Wolosker N, de Campos JRM, Kauffman P, et al. Evaluation of quality of life over time among 453 patients with hyperhidrosis submitted to endoscopic thoracic sympathectomy. J Vasc Surg 2012;55(1):154–6.
2. Lin TS, Wang NP, Huang LC. Pitfalls and complication avoidance associated with transthoracic endoscopic sympathectomy for primary hyperhidrosis (analysis of 2200 cases). Int J Surg Investig 2001; 2(5):377–85.
3. Lyra Rde M, Campos JR, Kang DW, et al. Guidelines for the prevention, diagnosis and treatment of compensatory hyperhidrosis. J Bras Pneumol 2008;34(11):967–77.
4. Sugimura H, Spratt EH, Compeau CG, et al. Thoracoscopic sympathetic clipping for hyperhidrosis: long-term results and reversibility. J Thorac

Cardiovasc Surg 2009;137(6):1370–6 [discussion: 1376–7].

5. Reisfeld R. Sympathectomy for hyperhidrosis: should we place the clamps at T2-T3 or T3-T4? Clin Auton Res 2006;16(6):384–9.

6. Dewey TM, Herbert MA, Hill SL, et al. One-year follow-up after thoracoscopic sympathectomy for hyperhidrosis: outcomes and consequences. Ann Thorac Surg 2006;81(4):1227–32 [discussion: 1232–3].

7. de Campos JRM, Wolosker N, Takeda FR, et al. The body mass index and level of resection: predictive factors for compensatory sweating after sympathectomy. Clin Auton Res 2005;15(2):116–20.

8. Li X, Tu Y-R, Lin M, et al. Endoscopic thoracic sympathectomy for palmar hyperhidrosis: a randomized control trial comparing T3 and T2-4 ablation. Ann Thorac Surg 2008;85(5):1747–51.

9. Yazbek G, Wolosker N, de Campos JRM, et al. Palmar hyperhidrosis–which is the best level of denervation using video-assisted thoracoscopic sympathectomy: T2 or T3 ganglion? J Vasc Surg 2005;42(2):281–5.

10. Kopelman D, Hashmonai M. The correlation between the method of sympathetic ablation for palmar hyperhidrosis and the occurrence of compensatory hyperhidrosis: a review. World J Surg 2008;32(11): 2343–56.

11. Cerfolio RJ, de Campos JRM, Bryant AS, et al. The Society of Thoracic Surgeons expert consensus for the surgical treatment of hyperhidrosis. Ann Thorac Surg 2011;91(5):1642–8.

12. Adson AW, Craig WM, Brown GE. Essential hyperhidrosis cured by sympathetic ganglionectomy and trunk resection. Arch Surg 1935; 31(5):794–806.

13. Chwajol M, Barrenechea IJ, Chakraborty S, et al. Impact of compensatory hyperhidrosis on patient satisfaction after endoscopic thoracic sympathectomy. Neurosurgery 2009;64(3):511–8 [discussion: 518].

14. Jeganathan R, Jordan S, Jones M, et al. Bilateral thoracoscopic sympathectomy: results and long-term follow-up. Interact Cardiovasc Thorac Surg 2008;7(1):67–70.

15. Schmidt J, Bechara FG, Altmeyer P, et al. Endoscopic thoracic sympathectomy for severe hyperhidrosis: impact of restrictive denervation on compensatory sweating. Ann Thorac Surg 2006; 81(3):1048–55.

16. Chiou TSM. Chronological changes of post-sympathectomy compensatory hyperhidrosis and recurrent sweating in patients with palmar hyperhidrosis. J Neurosurg Spine 2005;2(2):151–4.

17. Licht PB, Pilegaard HK. Severity of compensatory sweating after thoracoscopic sympathectomy. Ann Thorac Surg 2004;78(2):427–31.

18. Smidfelt K, Drott C. Late results of endoscopic thoracic sympathectomy for hyperhidrosis and facial blushing. Br J Surg 2011;98(12):1719–24.

19. Shoenfeld Y, Shapiro Y, Machtiger A, et al. Sweat studies in hyperhidrosis palmaris and plantaris. A survey of 60 patients before and after cervical sympathectomy. Dermatologica 1976;152(5):257–62.

20. Yang J, Tan J-J, Ye G-L, et al. T3/T4 thoracic sympathictomy and compensatory sweating in treatment of palmar hyperhidrosis. Chin Med J 2007;120(18): 1574–7.

21. Ray BS, Hinsey JC, Geohegan WA. Observations on the distribution of the sympathetic nerves to the pupil and upper extremity as determined by stimulation of the anterior roots in man. Ann Surg 1943;118(4): 647–55.

22. Chou S-H, Kao E-L, Lin C-C, et al. The importance of classification in sympathetic surgery and a proposed mechanism for compensatory hyperhidrosis: experience with 464 cases. Surg Endosc 2006; 20(11):1749–53.

23. Hashmonai M, Assalia A, Kopelman D. Thoracoscopic sympathectomy for palmar hyperhidrosis. Ablate or resect? Surg Endosc 2001;15(5): 435–41.

24. Fischel R, Cooper M, Kramer D. Microinvasive resectional sympathectomy using the harmonic scalpel. A more effective procedure with fewer side effects for treating essential hyperhidrosis of the hands, face or axillae. Clin Auton Res 2003; 13(Suppl 1):I66–70.

25. Gossot D, Galetta D, Pascal A, et al. Long-term results of endoscopic thoracic sympathectomy for upper limb hyperhidrosis. Ann Thorac Surg 2003;75(4): 1075–9.

26. Dumont P, Denoyer A, Robin P. Long-term results of thoracoscopic sympathectomy for hyperhidrosis. Ann Thorac Surg 2004;78(5):1801–7.

27. de Campos JRM, Kauffman P, Werebe E, et al. Quality of life, before and after thoracic sympathectomy: report on 378 operated patients. Ann Thorac Surg 2003;76(3):886–91.

28. Ishy A, de Campos JRM, Wolosker N, et al. Objective evaluation of patients with palmar hyperhidrosis submitted to two levels of sympathectomy: T3 and T4. Interact Cardiovasc Thorac Surg 2011;12(4): 545–8.

29. Munia MAS, Wolosker N, Kauffman P, et al. A randomized trial of T3-T4 versus T4 sympathectomy for isolated axillary hyperhidrosis. J Vasc Surg 2007;45(1):130–3.

30. Liu Y, Yang J, Liu J, et al. Surgical treatment of primary palmar hyperhidrosis: a prospective randomized study comparing T3 and T4 sympathicotomy. Eur J Cardiothorac Surg 2009;35(3):398–402.

31. Lecerf J-M, Reitz C, de Chasteigner A. Evaluation of discomfort and complications in a population of

18,102 patients overweight or obese patients. Presse Med 2003;2(15):689–95 [in French].

32. Panhofer P, Ringhofer C, Gleiss A, et al. Quality of life after sympathetic surgery at the T4 ganglion for primary hyperhidrosis: clip application versus diathermic cut. Int J Surg 2014;12(12):1478–83.

33. Hida K, Sakai T, Hayashi M, et al. Sympathotomy for palmar hyperhidrosis: the cutting versus clamping methods. Clin Auton Res 2015;25(5):271–6.

34. Kocher GJ, Taha A, Ahler M, et al. Is clipping the preferable technique to perform sympathicotomy? A retrospective study and review of the literature. Langenbecks Arch Surg 2015;400(1):107–12.

35. Findikcioglu A, Kilic D, Hatipoglu A. Is clipping superior to cauterization in the treatment of palmar hyperhidrosis? Thorac Cardiovasc Surg 2014;62(5):445–9.

36. Yanagihara TK, Ibrahimiye A, Harris C, et al. Analysis of clamping versus cutting of T3 sympathetic nerve for severe palmar hyperhidrosis. J Thorac Cardiovasc Surg 2010;140(5):984–9.

37. Reisfeld R, Nguyen R, Pnini A. Endoscopic thoracic sympathectomy for hyperhidrosis: experience with both cauterization and clamping methods. Surg Laparosc Endosc Percutan Tech 2002;12(4):255–67.

38. Steiner Z, Cohen Z, Kleiner O, et al. Do children tolerate thoracoscopic sympathectomy better than adults? Pediatr Surg Int 2008;24(3):343–7.

39. Coveliers H, Meyer M, Gharagozloo F, et al. Robotic selective postganglionic thoracic sympathectomy for the treatment of hyperhidrosis. Ann Thorac Surg 2013;95(1):269–74.

40. Bryant AS, Cerfolio RJ. Satisfaction and compensatory hyperhidrosis rates 5 years and longer after video-assisted thoracoscopic sympathotomy for hyperhidrosis. J Thorac Cardiovasc Surg 2014;147(4):1160–1.

41. Cladellas E, Callejas MA, Grimalt R. A medical alternative to the treatment of compensatory sweating. Dermatol Ther 2008;21(5):406–8.

42. Simpson LL. Identification of the major steps in botulinum toxin action. Annu Rev Pharmacol Toxicol 2004;44:167–93.

43. Jankovic J. Treatment of cervical dystonia with botulinum toxin. Mov Disord 2004;19(Suppl 8):S109–15.

44. Heckmann M, Ceballos-Baumann AO, Plewig G. Hyperhidrosis Study Group. Botulinum toxin A for axillary hyperhidrosis (excessive sweating). N Engl J Med 2001;344(7):488–93.

45. Naumann M, Lowe NJ. Botulinum toxin type A in treatment of bilateral primary axillary hyperhidrosis: randomised, parallel group, double blind, placebo controlled trial. BMJ 2001;323(7313):596–9.

46. Schnider P, Binder M, Auff E, et al. Double-blind trial of botulinum A toxin for the treatment of focal hyperhidrosis of the palms. Br J Dermatol 1997;136(4):548–52.

47. Lowe NJ, Yamauchi PS, Lask GP, et al. Efficacy and safety of botulinum toxin type a in the treatment of palmar hyperhidrosis: a double-blind, randomized, placebo-controlled study. Dermatol Surg 2002;28(9):822–7.

48. Kim WO, Kil HK, Yoon KB, et al. Botulinum toxin: a treatment for compensatory hyperhidrosis in the trunk. Dermatol Surg 2009;35(5):833–8 [discussion: 838].

49. Adefusika JA, Brewer JD. OnabotulinumtoxinA therapy for compensatory hyperhidrosis. J Cosmet Dermatol 2013;12(3):232–4.

50. Efthymiou CA, Thorpe JAC. Compensatory hyperhidrosis: a consequence of truncal sympathectomy treated by video assisted application of botulinum toxin and reoperation. Eur J Cardiothorac Surg 2008;33(6):1157–8.

51. Wolosker N, de Campos JR, Kauffman P, et al. An alternative to treat palmar hyperhidrosis: use of oxybutynin. Clin Auton Res 2011;21(6):389–93.

52. Wolosker N, Campos JR, Kauffman P, et al. The use of oxybutynin for treating facial hyperhidrosis. An Bras Dermatol 2011;86(3):451–6.

53. Wolosker N, Teivelis MP, Krutman M, et al. Long-term results of oxybutynin treatment for palmar hyperhidrosis. Clin Auton Res 2014;24(6):297–303.

54. Wolosker N, Teivelis MP, Krutman M, et al. Long-term results of oxybutynin use in treating facial hyperhidrosis. An Bras Dermatol 2014;89(6):912–6.

55. Walling HW, Swick BL. Treatment options for hyperhidrosis. Am J Clin Dermatol 2011;12(5):285–95.

56. Gong TK, Kim DW. Effectiveness of oral glycopyrrolate use in compensatory hyperhidrosis patients. Korean J Pain 2013;26(1):89–93.

57. Teivelis MP, Wolosker N, Krutman M, et al. Compensatory hyperhidrosis: results of pharmacologic treatment with oxybutynin. Ann Thorac Surg 2014;98(5):1797–802.

58. Karlsson-Groth A, Rystedt A, Swartling C. Treatment of compensatory hyperhidrosis after sympathectomy with botulinum toxin and anticholinergics. Clin Auton Res 2015;25(3):161–7.

59. Lin C-C, Mo LR, Lee LS, et al. Thoracoscopic T2-sympathetic block by clipping–a better and reversible operation for treatment of hyperhidrosis palmaris: experience with 326 cases. Eur J Surg Suppl 1998;580:13–6.

60. Telaranta T. Secondary sympathetic chain reconstruction after endoscopic thoracic sympathicotomy. Eur J Surg Suppl 1998;580:17–8.

# Less Common Side Effects of Sympathetic Surgery

Lyall A. Gorenstein, MD[a], Mark J. Krasna, MD[b],*

## KEYWORDS

- Endoscopic thoracic sympathectomy • Complications • Morbidity • Autonomic function
- Side effects of ETS

## KEY POINTS

- Endoscopic thoracic sympathectomy (ETS) is a highly effective surgical procedure for patients with severe palmar hyperhidrosis.
- Because of the elective nature of this procedure, safe performance of ETS is imperative.
- Although it is a relatively straightforward procedure, intraoperative complications can occur, especially if thoracic anatomy is not well-understood.
- Patient selection and surgical accuracy are imperative for reproducible results with high patient satisfaction.
- Certain side effects of ETS are well-known and patients must be informed of these.

## INTRODUCTION

Video-assisted thoracic sympathectomy also known as endoscopic thoracic sympathectomy (ETS), is a well-established, effective therapy for patients with severe palmar hyperhidrosis that is refractory to medical therapy. ETS has been shown to effectively eliminate palmar hyperhidrosis, while improving quality of life and reducing associated social anxiety.[1–3] Before the development of endoscopic thoracic techniques in the late 1980s, thoracic sympathectomy for palmar hyperhidrosis was rarely performed. Minimally invasive thoracic techniques, which evolved through the 1990s, facilitate performance of thoracic sympathectomies with minimal surgical trauma and led to the widespread acceptance of ETS for patients with palmar hyperhidrosis.[4]

Despite its effectiveness in eliminating palmar hyperhidrosis and widespread use, there are many variations of the ETS technique, especially with regard to trocar placement, lung isolation, exposure of the sympathetic nerve, and the type of and location of surgical sympathectomy. These technical variations, in addition to physiologic side effects of sympathectomy such as compensatory sweating, have resulted in significant controversy with regard to the role of ETS in the overall management of patients with palmar hyperhidrosis.

It is, therefore, imperative that ETS be performed safely, without surgical complications so that the benefits are not overshadowed by either side effects or long-term complications. In this paper, we review the more common early and late potential complications of ETS and offer our recommendations for avoidance, based on our personal experience, having performed thousands of ETS procedures over several decades (**Box 1**).

## INTRAOPERATIVE COMPLICATIONS
### Lung Isolation

To perform ETS, lung isolation is generally required. This can be achieved either by placing a double-lumen tube, or creating a unilateral pneumothorax with $CO_2$ insufflation. Both techniques are equally effective, with specific advantages and disadvantages inherent with each, and

a New York Presbyterian Hospital, Columbia University, 161 Fort Washington Avenue, New York, NY 10032, USA; b Meridian Cancer Care, Rutgers-Robert Wood Johnson Medical School, Jersey Shore University Medical Center, Ackerman South rm 553, 1945 rt 33, Neptune, NJ 07753, USA
* Corresponding author.
E-mail address: MKrasna@meridianhealth.com

Thorac Surg Clin 26 (2016) 453–458
http://dx.doi.org/10.1016/j.thorsurg.2016.06.010
1547-4127/16/© 2016 Elsevier Inc. All rights reserved.

---

**Box 1**
**Complications of endoscopic thoracic sympathectomy**

*Intraoperative*
- Failure to obtain adequate lung isolation
- Bleeding
- Pneumothorax
- Incomplete sympathectomy
- Inaccurate or wrong level sympathectomy
- Phrenic nerve injury
- Aorta or great vessel injury
- Thoracic duct injury

*Early postoperative*
- Pneumothorax
- Hemothorax
- Intercostal neuralgia
- Chest pain/pleuritis
- Horner's syndrome

*Late postoperative*
- Intercostal neuralgia
- Cardiac
- Recurrent symptoms of palmar hyperhidrosis

---

therefore the choice of technique is surgeon specific. Although this author personally has moved away from using a double-lumen endotracheal tube for a routine ETS procedure, in patients who had a prior intrathoracic procedure, where there may be significant pleural adhesions, a double-lumen tube could be advantageous. Excellent visualization of the upper thorax and the sympathetic trunk are obtained by insufflating $CO_2$ at 10 mm Hg pressure (not to exceed), without impacting venous return or hemodynamics. Frequent blood pressure measurements are necessary while insufflating $CO_2$, especially when the patient's head is elevated, because venous return can be impaired; however, we do not routinely use an arterial line.

Pleural adhesions are uncommon in this patient population, but on occasion will be encountered. Depending on the severity adhesions, an extra port may be required to provide countertraction on the lung while dividing adhesions. Care must be used to not only avoid visceral pleural injury, but also be aware of the regional anatomy so as to avoid injury to the aorta, esophagus, subclavian vessels, phrenic nerve, or stellate ganglion. If major adhesions are divided, leaving a small pleural chest tube connected to pleural drainage while the contralateral sympathectomy is performed will avoid hemodynamic instability if there is undetected visceral injury and a small air leak.

## Unusual Anatomy

Most patients undergoing ETS for palmar hyperhidrosis are young and healthy, without medical or pulmonary comorbidities. On occasion, however, unexpected anatomy can be encountered. The most common is an azygous lobe, found on the right upper lobe. Reported incidence is 1% of population. When encountered, the pleural mesentery needs to be opened immediately superior to the azygous vein to expose the sympathetic trunk. The azygous vein does not impair exposing the sympathetic trunk, or completion of the sympathectomy, and can be left intact. After completion of the sympathectomy, the azygous lobe does not need to placed behind the pleural mesentery when the lung reexpands.

Rarely, an asymptomatic apical bleb or bulla can be encountered, especially when performing ETS on teenage or young adult males. The natural history asymptomatic apical blebs or bulla is not known. On 2 occasions, this author has chosen to resect asymptomatic bullae from the lung apex. If a bleb or bulla is not removed, the anesthesiologist should be mindful during lung reexpansion not to hyperinflate the lung.

## Pneumothorax

Inadvertent lung injury can occur when inserting a Veress needle, trocars, or lysing adhesions. This may only become apparent when the contralateral sympathectomy is being performed resulting in unexplained hypotension. If a contralateral tension pneumothorax is suspected, $CO_2$ insufflation should be discontinued immediately and a chest tube inserted on the contralateral side. Once the pneumothorax has been treated then the sympathectomy can be completed safely.

There are many different techniques to evacuate $CO_2$ from the pleural space. However, it is not uncommon to see a very small apical pneumothorax on the immediate postoperative chest radiograph. Provided it is small, no further treatment is required, because $CO_2$ is absorbed relatively rapidly from the pleural space. We generally evacuate the pace with a small chest tube (12 Fr) and remove it while the anesthetist is administering a large positive pressure breath. Of those persistent pneumothorax cases, fewer than 10% require a chest tube, and few of those require overnight drainage.

## Bleeding

Significant intraoperative bleeding during thoracic sympathectomy is rare. When it does occur, it usually emanates from the intercostal vessels either during trocar placement, or during dissection of the sympathetic nerve.

There are many different techniques described with regard to trocar size, and placements. Some surgeons employee a single port technique, which typically requires using a 10-mm trocar or greater, and may have a greater propensity to injure the intercostal vessels. This author prefers the 2-port technique, using either 3- or 5-mm trocars, which may reduce the risk of intercostal vessel or nerve injury. Other authors uses a pediatric reusable metal trocar, which is 8 mm, with a small operating scope and working channel for 2- to 5-mm instruments.

When bleeding occurs during the dissection and mobilization of the sympathetic nerve, it usually is from the intercostal vein or artery. Depending on the nature of the injury, compression with an endoscopic peanut usually is sufficient to achieve hemostasis, and rarely will the vessel need to be isolated and clipped. On the right side, the uppermost intercostal veins join the azygous vein just proximal to its junction with the superior vena cava. Injury to any of those intercostal veins can result in significant bleeding from the azygous vein and therefore prompt control with external pressure, and exposure is necessary, to facilitate placing Hemoclips. Attempting to cauterize can often exacerbate the bleeding.

When performing a sympathectomy above the superior aspect of the second rib, the subclavian artery can be injured. Achieving rapid control of the injury is necessary, while adequate exposure and proximal control of the vessel is obtained. Injury to the aorta, great vessels, or the subclavian vein can occur when dividing adhesions, when a fused pleural space is encountered, and when anatomic landmarks are distorted or obscured; therefore, a clear understanding of the thoracoscopic anatomy is key to avoiding these complications.

## Incomplete Sympathectomy

Although there is no agreed upon technique of ETS for palmar hyperhidrosis among surgeons, when performing thoracic sympathectomy or ETS for palmar hyperhidrosis, it is essential that every surgeon be consistent in their procedure from patient to patient. This requires using consistent anatomic landmarks to identify the thoracic sympathetic nerve. Failure to identify the anatomy correctly could result in performing the sympathectomy at the incorrect level, resulting in failure to eliminate palmar hyperhidrosis, or complications such as Horner's syndrome or severe compensatory sweating.

A potential advantage of clamping versus cutting is that the Hemoclip, which can be seen on a routine chest radiograph, provides documentation as to the level of the sympathectomy.[5–8]

This author prefers to use the subclavian artery and its relationship to the first rib, to then to identify the second and third ribs. This is far more consistent than relying on the venous anatomy or other structures.

Similarly, it is essential to open the posterior parietal pleura, which cover the sympathetic nerve before either cutting or clipping the interganglionic segment. Videos exist whereby a Hemoclip is placed on the sympathetic nerve without opening the pleura, only to have the clip dislodge. Opening the pleura to place the clip or encircling the chain before cautery division again avoids incomplete division of the nerve. Parallel branches and chains should be identified.

## POSTOPERATIVE COMPLICATIONS
### Pleural Complications

Because ETS is such a safe procedure, in most centers it is performed as an outpatient procedure, with patients being discharged several hours postoperatively. Institutions tend to develop their own postoperative protocols regarding observation time, postoperative laboratory studies, and chest radiographs before discharge.

We perform a chest radiograph when the patient arrives in the recovery room. It is not uncommon to have small residual apical pneumothoraces, which generally do not need any intervention. This author does not routinely obtain follow-up chest radiographs before discharge. Similarly, there may be some subcutaneous emphysema at the port sites, which also is benign and needs no treatment. Both postoperative pneumothorax and subcutaneous emphysema can be minimized if a thorough attempt is made to evacuate $CO_2$ from the pleural space before port removal.

Patients often complain of some pleuritic type chest pain after bilateral ETS. We believe it emanates from either opening the pleura adjacent to the sympathetic nerve or from baroreceptors on the visceral pleura of the lung. It is usually self-limiting and dissipates over several days after surgery. Rarely, this pain can be from the trocar port placement. We generally do not prescribe narcotic analgesics after this surgery, having found that either acetaminophen or nonsteroidal antiinflammatory drugs suffice.

A pleural effusion on the postoperative chest radiograph could represent blood in the pleural space, which will mandate ongoing observation and possible intervention if it seems to be increasing, or if the patient is symptomatic. Rare case of chylothorax has been described.[9]

### Postoperative Pain

Intercostal neuralgia can occur after any thoracoscopic procedure. This type of pain typically occurs because of either the location of port placement, using large trocars in patients with narrow intercostal spaces, or from compression of the intercostal nerve by the trocar during the surgical procedure. This complication is very rare in our experience after ETS. The 2-port technique with either 3- or 5-mm trocars helps to minimize the incidence of intercostal neuralgia. Unless the intercostal nerve is injured during exposure of the sympathetic nerve or during clamp placement across the sympathetic nerve, intercostal neuralgia from the port sites is usually self-limiting, and subsides spontaneously.

### Horner's Syndrome

Most surgeons, when performing ETS for palmar hyperhidrosis, avoid the stellate ganglion, which lies between the first and second ribs. If the sympathetic nerve is manipulated above the superior aspect of the second rib, the stellate ganglion can be traumatized resulting in a Horner syndrome. When ETS was first described, the sympathectomy often begun on the superior aspect of the second rib, and the reported incidence of Horner's syndrome was approximately 1%. Because most surgeons currently perform either T3 or T4 sympathectomy for palmar hyperhidrosis, the incidence of Horner's syndrome is negligible. Failure to identify the anatomy correctly may result in inadvertent division of the sympathetic nerve near the stellate ganglion.

ETS for facial blushing remains controversial. When ETS is performed for this indication, care must be taken when dissecting on the sympathetic nerve above the second rib, avoiding traction on the nerve and avoiding electrocautery in and around the sympathetic nerve, which can injure the stellate ganglion because of the capacity for conduction of electricity by nerve tissue.

### Cardiac

The long-term cardiovascular effects of bilateral thoracoscopic sympathectomy for hyperhidrosis and its effect on exercise tolerance are poorly understood, and contradictory. Papa and colleagues[10] studied the cardiovascular impact of bilateral T2/T3 transsupraclavicular sympathectomy performed for hyperhidrosis in 39 patients aged 17 to 34 years. Resting heart rate and systolic blood pressure were reduced both at rest and with exercise at 30 days postoperatively, and remained so at 2 years, indicating a β-blocker–type impact on cardiac sympathetic tone. Drott and colleagues[11] selected 18 patients at random from their cohort of 535 patients undergoing elective bilateral endoscopic electro cautery of the upper thoracic sympathetic ganglia (T2-T4), to undergo cycle ergometer test before and after surgery. No impairment of physical working capacity was reported. Noppen and colleagues[12] studied 13 consecutive patients aged 14 to 44 years before and after T2/T3 thoracoscopic sympathicolysis, and reported a reduction in heart rate with rest and with maximal exercise, but no impairment of exercise capacity or cardiorespiratory response to exercise. Wehrwein and coworkers[13] measured a variety of cardiovascular and hemodynamic parameters in patients with hyperhidrosis, both before and after ETS, concluding that ETS had no impact on either $mVO_2$ or exercise tolerance. Schmidt and associates[14] measured the impact of T2 ETS on cardiac parameters, comparing matched controlled patients with and without hyperhidrosis, concluding that ETS returned cardiac autonomic response toward baseline. The observations and conclusions of these studies are limited because of the small sample sizes and the variability of the sympathetic technique used. There are many large series of ETS wherein there are no cardiac complications reported.[1,2,4,15]

Autonomic sympathetic innervation of the heart is predominantly from sympathetic fibers that arise from the stellate ganglion, and course medially. Sympathetic procedures that use electrocautery to divide the sympathetic chain and surrounding adjacent tissue along the superior aspect of the second rib are likely going to disturb these microscopic branches (**Fig. 1**). Whereas procedures that isolate the sympathetic nerve precisely either on the second rib when performing T2 sympathectomy or more distally with either T3/T4 sympathectomy are less likely to disrupt these branches. Variability in both surgical techniques and anatomy of the sympathetic innervation of the heart may account for this rarely observed side effect of ETS.

### Patient Satisfaction

Although severe palmar hyperhidrosis can be quite debilitating, impacting all aspects of daily life for those affected, ETS epitomizes an elective surgical procedure. It is imperative that ETS be performed safely without any serious perioperative morbidity and absolutely no mortality, and it is essential that long-term outcomes meet patient's expectations. Achieving high patient satisfaction depends on several factors, including patient selection and preoperative education.

## Patient Selection

Achieving good results from ETS begins with selecting ideal candidates. Patient satisfaction from ETS, when performed for palmar hyperhidrosis is generally quite good, with some moderate variability. However, for other types of hyperhidrosis, the results are less uniform and we believe that only patients with severe symptoms based on the hyperhidrosis severity scale and are refractory to medical therapy should undergo ETS. Patients with diffuse hyperhidrosis, medical comorbidities, or depressive disorders are likely to be disappointed after ETS.

## Preoperative Education

Patient satisfaction after ETS is profoundly impacted by their expectations. Therefore, it is critical to educate patients before surgery about the expected results in regard to relief of palmar,

plantar, and axillary hyperhidrosis. It is especially important to emphasize potential complications of ETS and predictable side effects, such as compensatory sweating, during the preoperative evaluation.

## Standardized Surgical Procedure

There remains great controversy as to which ETS procedure achieves the best results for patients with palmar hyperhidrosis. Only a well-designed multiinstitutional international randomized trial will settle this issue. Because a study of that magnitude is very challenging to perform, it behooves each surgeon who performs ETS, to standardize the procedure they perform for patients with palmar hyperhidrosis, so that their results are reproducible and consistent.

## Evaluation of Personal Surgical Results

Along with standardizing the ETS procedure, it is essential that each surgeon evaluate his or her results postoperatively. There are several commonly used questionnaires available to assess patient satisfaction and long-term results after ETS. We generally assess patient satisfaction at 1 year after ETS. Ongoing collection and assessment of these data is laborious but essential for patient education when they are deciding to proceed with ETS.

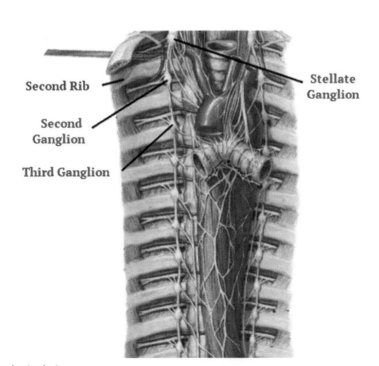

**Fig. 1.** The sympathetic chain.

## REFERENCES

1. Kwong KF, Cooper LB, Bennett LA, et al. Clinical experience in 397 consecutive thoracoscopic sympathectomies. Ann Thorac Surg 2005;80:1063–6.
2. Lin TS, Fang HY. Transthoracic endoscopic sympathectomy in the treatment of palmar hyperhidrosis-with emphasis on perioperative management (1,360 case analyses). Surg Neurol 1999;52:453–7.
3. Schneier FR, Heimberg RG, Liebowitz MR, et al. Social anxiety and functional impairment in patients seeking surgical evaluation for hyperhidrosis. Compr Psychiatry 2012;53:1181–6.
4. Zacherl J, Imhof M, Huber ER, et al. Video assistance reduces complication rate of thoracoscopic sympathectomy for hyperhidrosis. Ann Thorac Surg 1999;68:1177–81.
5. Sugimura H, Spratt EH, Compeau CG, et al. Thoracoscopic sympathetic clipping for hyperhidrosis: long-term results and reversibility. J Thorac Cardiovasc Surg 2009;137:1370–8.
6. Panhofer P, Ringhofer C, Gleiss A, et al. Quality of life after surgery at the T4 ganglion for primary hyperhidrosis: clip application versus diathermic cut. Int J Surg 2014;12:1478–83.
7. Smidfelt K, Drott C. Late results of endoscopic thoracic sympathectomy for hyperhidrosis and facial blushing. Br J Surg 2012;98:1719–24.
8. Yanagihara TK, Ibrahimiye A, Harris C. Analysis of clamping versus cutting of T3 sympathetic nerve for severe palmar hyperhidrosis. J Thorac Cardiovasc Surg 2010;140:984–9.
9. Gossot D. Chylothorax after endoscopic thoracic sympathectomy. Surg Endosc 1996;10(9):949.
10. Papa MZ, Schneiderman J, Tucker EBN, et al. Cardiovascular changes after bilateral upper dorsal sympathectomy. Short and long-term effects. Ann Surg 1986;204:715–8.
11. Drott C, Claes G, Gothberg G, et al. Cardiac effects of endoscopic electrocautery of the upper thoracic sympathetic chain. Eur J Surg Suppl 1994;(572):65–70.
12. Noppen M, Dendale P, Hagers Y, et al. Changes in cardiocirculatory autonomic function after thoracoscopic upper dorsal sympathicolysis for essential hyperhidrosis. J Auton Nerv Syst 1996;60:115–20.
13. Wehrwein EA, Schmidt JE, Elvebak RL, et al. Hemodynamics following endoscopic thoracic sympathotomy for palmar hyperhidrosis. Clin Auton Res 2011;21(1):3–10.
14. Schmidt JE, Wehrwein EA, Gronbach LA, et al. Autonomic function following endoscopic thoracic sympathotomy for hyperhidrosis. Clin Auton Res 2011;21(1):7–11.
15. Cerfolio RJ, Milanez de Campos JR, Bryant AS, et al. The Society of Thoracic Surgeons expert consensus for the surgical treatment of hyperhidrosis. Ann Thorac Surg 2011;91:1642–8.

# Facial Blushing
## Patient Selection and Long-Term Results

Smidfelt Kristian, MD[a], Drott Christer, MD, PhD[b,c],*

**KEYWORDS**

- Facial blushing • ETS • Sympathectomy • Social phobia

**KEY POINTS**

- Facial blushing may have a severe negative impact on the quality of life.
- The first line of treatment should be psychological and/or pharmacologic.
- If nonsurgical treatments fail, upper thoracic sympathetic denervation may yield rewarding results.
- Side effects (mainly severe sweating on the trunk of the body) of surgical treatment may be severe and cause the patient to regret the procedure.
- Patient satisfaction with the outcome of surgery decreases over time.

## INTRODUCTION

Redness of the face may have many underlying causes.[1] This article deals only with the type of rapid onset facial blushing triggered by psychological stimuli. It typically peaks within seconds and subsides within minutes when the triggering event has passed. Blushing under certain circumstances is quite normal, and is mediated by increased sympathetic nervous signaling causing cutaneous vasodilatation.[2] Charles Darwin in 1872 described facial blushing "as the most peculiar and the most human of all expressions of emotions" and that it is "the thinking about what other people think of us which excites a blush."[3]

Facial blushing in embarrassing situations is present in all cultures.[4] It has also been shown that blushing has a remedial value (sympathy, trustworthiness) in people watching actors who blush by mishaps and transgression.[5] Blushing is thus an adequate social signal; however, when very easily triggered and severe, it may cause avoidance of social interaction and have severe and negative impact on the quality of daily life.[6]

It is unclear why some individuals live in fear of blushing, which may dominate their social life, whereas others regard it as a minor nuisance, not requiring any treatment, and some disregard it completely.

Facial blushing is often present in social anxiety disorders (SAD) and regarded as the hallmark of embarrassment.[7] Facial blushing has also been described as a specific symptom of social phobia not associated with other forms of anxiety disorders.[4] SAD patients with blushing seem to be a distinct subgroup compared with those without a blushing problem.[8] It is unclear whether SAD with blushing is a primary SAD subtype or a secondary SAD owing to blushing.[9] The prevalence of blushing is unknown, but around 50% of patients with social phobia blush frequently.[10] Social phobia is a common psychiatric disorder with prevalence rates of around 10%.[11,12]

The first report on sympathetic ablation for facial blushing appeared in 1985.[13] These authors' experience with treating facial blushing started in the early 1990s when several patients who had

Disclosure: The authors have nothing to disclose.
<sup>a</sup> Department of Vascular Surgery, Sahlgrenska University Hospital, Per Dubbsgatan 1, Gothenburg S-41345, Sweden; <sup>b</sup> Borås Hospital, Brämhultsvägen 53, Borås S-50182, Sweden; <sup>c</sup> Sahlgrenska University, Gothenburg, Sweden
* Corresponding author. Sahlgrenska University, Gothenburg, Sweden.
E-mail address: christer.drott@vgregion.se

Thorac Surg Clin 26 (2016) 459–463
http://dx.doi.org/10.1016/j.thorsurg.2016.06.011
1547-4127/16/© 2016 Elsevier Inc. All rights reserved.

undergone endoscopic thoracic sympathetic (ETS) denervation for palmar hyperhidrosis reported great satisfaction of being rid of their facial blushing as well as their sweating. We then started to offer ETS to patients with social anxiety and facial blushing as a dominant symptom in cooperation with a psychiatrist specialized in social phobia treatment. We were warned initially by the psychiatrist that the social phobia might persist and focus be turned from facial redness to some other symptom. This was, however, not the case and the early excellent results were reported in the first comprehensive study of surgical treatment for facial blushing.[6] Previous reports had consisted of small series, which superficially reported "positive" results in a majority of patients.[13–15]

For obvious reasons, people with social phobia and facial blushing do not readily demand treatment, because this would provoke their very problem. Instead, most patients have developed an avoidance behavior to situations likely to trigger their blushing. This often means that they exclude themselves not only from social interactions, but also from professions that they otherwise would prefer. When they finally decide to seek professional advice, they are often met by doctors who are unaware of the impact of severe facial blushing on the quality of life, and trivialization is common. Many patients have been addressed with expressions like "it is cute to blush," "you will get used to it," or "do not bother about it" by medical professionals. By not treating these patients' concerns seriously, doctors inflict further trauma to an already fragile patient population.

## NONSURGICAL TREATMENT

Nonsurgical treatment should be the first line of treatment. Selective serotonin reuptake inhibitors have beneficial effects, reducing facial blushing and social phobia.[16–18] Beta-receptor blockers may reduce blushing, but scientific support is lacking.[19] An experimental study supported that topical ibuprofen gel application may reduce facial reddening in provoked embarrassment and aerobic exercise, but further research is required before any clinical recommendation can be made.[20]

Psychological treatment such as cognitive–behavioral therapy has been used extensively with good results in social phobia, although few studies have addressed the blushing phenomenon specifically.[18] Psychological treatments are usually considered time consuming, but even a weekend therapy with attention training and behavioral therapy have beneficial effects on the fear of blushing.[21]

## SURGICAL TREATMENT AND PATIENT SELECTION

Before selecting patients for surgery, the surgeon should be selected. Adequate experience in thoracoscopy and the capacity to deal with intraoperative complications is mandatory. Previous pleural disease or thoracotomy may cause adhesions precluding endoscopic access to the upper thoracic sympathetic chain. Although there is no consensus on the extent and level of sympathetic ablation, most surgeons include the level of the second rib, so access to the upper part of the thoracic cavity is required.[22]

The authors believe that patient selection is a misnomer and that the surgeon should guide the patient to an informed and wise selection of treatment by thorough disclosure of all the pros and cons of ETS. Efforts should be made to ensure that the patient have realistic expectations of the beneficial effects of surgery. Even if the facial blushing is abolished, it often takes time to alter a social avoidance behavior and sometimes further psychological counseling is required.

The facial blushing should have a severe impact on the quality of daily life. The social fear should be linked overwhelmingly to their blushing. The only kind of blushing that responds very well to ETS is the facial, rapid onset type that appears within seconds and is associated with profound feelings of embarrassment and an intense urge to flee from the situation that triggered it. In our experience, ETS works poorly on more slowly emerging facial redness as well as on upper chest and neck blushing. We have had several patients with a mixture of blushing types reporting excellent effect on the rapid onset and poor or no effect on the other types of blushing. Pharmacologic and psychological treatment regimens should fail before surgical treatment options are considered. Thorough disclosure of complications and side effects are mandatory, especially the risk of severe compensatory sweating and regret of the procedure. Age has been reported as a predictor of satisfaction; younger patients were more satisfied than older.[23] We could not confirm this effect, because age was not correlated with the effect of surgery or overall satisfaction.[24] Regarding side effects, men suffered more from compensatory sweating than women and the impact of compensatory sweating on daily living decreased significantly with age.[24] Overall satisfaction rates reflects a combination of the effects and side effects of surgery where women are more satisfied than men.[24] The authors believe that patients should be encouraged to search the Internet for information but be warned about exaggerated, both positive and negative, testimonials.

Open surgical upper thoracic sympathetic denervation is obsolete nowadays. The endoscopic approach permits bilateral procedures in the same operation setting. The insufflation of carbon dioxide into the pleural cavity permits single lumen endotracheal intubation. The sympathetic nerve traffic may be abolished by various methods such as resection, cutting or clipping but the result will be the same.

Regardless of sympathetic denervation methods, patients must be informed that ETS should be regarded as irreversible.[25]

## Complications

Surgical complications are rare when ETS is performed by an experienced surgeon. Pneumothorax requiring chest drainage is not a severe complication, but is reported in up to 10% of patients.[26] Damage to somatic nerves, mainly intercostal nerves, depends on the operative technique and diameter of the instruments. In most publications this is rare but persisting pain has been reported in up to 8% of patients.[26] Damage to the stellate ganglion may occur as a result of thermal damage, nerve traction, or miscalculation of the target ganglion. The ensuing Horner's eye syndrome may vary from 0% to 4%.[26] Occasionally, asymmetrical denervation may give rise to a Harlequin phenomenon (one-half of the face still red and the other one-half pale). This requires a redo procedure on the still blushing side. The most dangerous complication is intrathoracic bleeding, which has even been fatal.[27,28] Readiness for thoracotomy and control of bleeding is mandatory. Our group has performed more than 4000 ETS procedures without ever needing conversion to an open thoracotomy. We have had 1, previously unpublished, postoperative death 12 years ago. It was a 32-year-old, previously healthy woman who underwent an uneventful ETS procedure and postoperative recovery. She was back on the ward, fully awake and telephoned her husband that she felt well. Six hours postoperatively she was found with cardiac arrest without having pressed the alarm button beside her. Forensic autopsy failed to find the cause of death and there was no sign of bleeding or other surgical complication.

## Side Effects

Upper thoracic sympathetic denervation inhibits the sweating on the upper part of the body. The main side effect is increased sweating on the rest of the body, often called "compensatory sweating." The mechanism behind this is quite obscure; it can be profuse despite no need for body temperature regulation. Depending on the definition, the prevalence of compensatory sweating has been reported in 10%[29] to 98%[30] of patients after ETS. The main reason for regretting the ETS procedure is severe compensatory sweating. Regret rates have been reported at between 0% (which is hardly credible) and 15.5%.[24,31] Gustatory sweating is triggered by ingestion of different, often spicy, food or drinks, which results in increased sweating mainly in the face. The pathophysiology behind this phenomenon is poorly understood. Gustatory sweating has been reported in around one-third of patients.[31,32] The upper thoracic sympathetic chain innervates the heart and denervation results in a partial cardiac "beta-blockade."[33] This results in the relative bradycardia noticed by many patients as fewer heart palpitations in mentally stressful situations.[6] A lower sympathetic drive on the heart is also beneficial for cardiac diseases such as certain dysrhythmias[34] and angina pectoris.[35] Concerns have been raised that physical performance might be impaired but cycle ergometer test before and after ETS showed no deterioration of work performance.[36] Cold hands are probably owing to denervation hypersensitivity of adrenergic receptors to circulating catecholamines, with a reported prevalence of around 1.5%.[24]

Complications and side effects after ETS seem to be the same regardless of indication.[24,27]

## LONG-TERM RESULTS OF SURGERY

Short- and mid-term results of ETS for facial blushing are excellent.[22,37] In 2011, our group published a report of 648 patients with facial blushing who were operated from 1989 to 1998 with a mean follow-up of 14.6 years.[24] We had a primary failure rate (patients not satisfied with the effect on blushing) of 14%. Most of those patients had predominantly slowly emerging facial and neck blushing. In the beginning, we were not aware of the poor effect on those types of blushing. Overall 73.5% of patients were satisfied to some degree with the outcome, whereas 11% were dissatisfied and 15.5% regretted the ETS. Women were significantly more satisfied than men despite there being no difference in effect. The explanation lies in the higher prevalence of compensatory sweating (85.4% in men vs 76.2% in women). Age was not correlated with effect or satisfaction rate. Improved quality of life was indicated by 72% of all patients. The view that satisfaction with surgery is related to the severity of perceived preoperative symptoms is supported by our long-term follow-up. Non- Scandinavian patients had the discomfort of long traveling and higher costs than Scandinavian patients. Those hurdles presumably led to a selection of patients with more severe symptoms and resulted in a very high satisfaction rate in this group.

A cohort of patients in this survey had answered a previous questionnaire after a mean follow-up of 3.7 years. The regret rate almost doubled between 3.7 years and 14.6 years of follow-up. Similarly, the overall satisfaction rate decreased by 8% over the interval. An explanation might be that 15% more of the respondents reported severe or incapacitating compensatory sweating between the surveys. Coveliers and colleagues[26] have reported long-term results in 26 patients where satisfaction rate decreased from 81% in short follow-up to 42% after a mean of 7.75 years. Our hypothesis for the reason of the decline in satisfaction rate and increased regret rate over time is that the side effects persist, whereas the memory of the suffering from blushing before surgery fades with time.

## SUMMARY

Facial blushing is not merely a cosmetic problem, but may have a severe negative impact on the quality of life. The National Institute for Health and Care Excellence guidelines recommends pharmacologic and psychological (cognitive–behavioral therapy) interventions before considering the surgical option with ETS.[38] We do agree that ETS should be used only in severe and incapacitating facial blushing that has been refractory to other treatments even if patients demand the "quick fix of surgery." Future research should be aimed at establishing predictors to identify patients with low risk of severe side effects and high likelihood of experiencing good effect on the blushing.

## REFERENCES

1. Izikson L, English JC 3rd, Zirwas MJ. The flushing patient: differential diagnosis, workup and treatment. J Am Acad Dermatol 2006;55:193–208.
2. Drummond PD, Lance JW. Facial flushing and sweating mediated by the sympathetic nervous system. Brain 1987;110:793–803.
3. Darwin C. The expression of the emotions in man and animals. In: Porter DM, Graham PW, editors. The portable Darwin. New York: Penguin books; 1993. p. 364–93.
4. Crozier WR. Social psychological perspectives on shyness, embarrassment and shame. In: Crozier WT, editor. Shyness and embarrassment.

5. Dijk C, de Jong PJ, Peters ML. The remedial value of blushing in the context of transgressions and mishaps. Emotion 2009;9(2):287–91.
6. Drott C, Claes G, Olsson-Rex L, et al. Successful treatment of facial blushing by endoscopic transthoracic sympathicotomy. Br J Dermatol 1998;138:639–43.
7. Buss AH. Self-consciousness and social anxiety. San Francisco (CA): Freeman; 1980.
8. Voncken MJ, Bögels SM. Physiological blushing in social anxiety disorder patients with and without blushing complaints: two subtypes? Biol Psychol 2009;81:86–94.
9. Pelissolo A, Moukheiber A, Lobjoie MA, et al. Is there a place for fear of blushing in social anxiety spectrum? Depress Anxiety 2012;29:62–70.
10. Amies PL, Gelder MG, Shaw PM. Social phobia: a comparative clinical study. Br J Psychiatry 1983;142:174–9.
11. Wacker HR, Mullejans R, Klein KH, et al. Identification of cases of anxiety disorders and affective disorders in the community according to the ICD-10 and DSM-III-R using the composite international diagnostic interview (CIDI). Int J Meth Psychiatr Res 1992;2:91–100.
12. Kessler RC, McGonagle KA, Zhao S, et al. Lifetime and 12-month prevalence of DSM-III-R psychiatric disorders in the United States: results from the National Comorbidity Survey. Arch Gen Psychiatry 1994;51:8–19.
13. Wittmoser R. Treatment of sweating and blushing by endoscopic surgery. Acta Neurochir (Wien) 1985;74:153–4.
14. Wepf R. Operative treatment of erythrophobia. Br J Surg 1993;80(Suppl):S95.
15. Julius AJ, van Mourik JC. Transaxillaire thoracale sympathectomie ter behandeling van primaire hyperhidrosis en rubeosis. Ned Tijdschr Geneeskd 1985;129:1042–5.
16. Connor KM, Davidson JR, Chung H, et al. Multidimensional effects of sertraline in social anxiety disorder. Depress Anxiety 2006;23:6–10.
17. Jadresic E, Súarez C, Palacios E, et al. Evaluating the efficacy of endoscopic thoracic sympathectomy for generalized social anxiety disorder with blushing complaints: a comparison with sertraline and no treatment- Santiago de Chile 2003-2009. Innov Clin Neurosci 2011;8:24–35.
18. Fahlén T. Social phobia: symptomatology and changes during drug treatment. Doctorial thesis. Department of Clinical Neuroscience. Section of Psychiatry and Neurochemistry. Gothenburg (Sweden): Goteborg University; 1995.
19. Drott C. Results of endoscopic thoracic sympathectomy (ETS) on hyperhidrosis, facial blushing, angina

Cambridge (UK): Cambridge University Press; 1990. p. 19–58.

pectoris, vascular disorders and pain syndromes of the hand and arm. Clin Auton Res 2003;13(Suppl 1): I26–30.

20. Drummond PD, Minosora K, Little G, et al. Topical ibuprofen inhibits blushing during embarrassment and facial flushing during aerobic exercise in people with a fear of blushing. Eur Neuropsychopharmacol 2013;23:1747–53.

21. Chaker S, Hofmann SG, Hoyer J. Can a one-weekend group therapy reduce fear of blushing. Results of an open trial. Anxiety Stress Coping 2010; 23:303–18.

22. Licht PB, Pilegaard HK, Ladegaard L. Sympathicotomy for isolated facial blushing: a randomized clinical trial. Ann Thorac Surg 2012;94:401–5.

23. Bell D, Jedynak J, Bell R. Predictors of outcome following endoscopic thoracic sympathectomy. ANZ J Surg 2014;84:68–72.

24. Smidfelt K, Drott C. Late results of endoscopic thoracic sympathectomy for hyperhidrosis and facial blushing. Br J Surg 2011;98:1719–24.

25. Schick CH, Bischof G, Cameron AA, et al. Sympathetic chain clipping for hyperhidrosis is not a reversible procedure. Surg Endosc 2013;27:3043.

26. Coveliers H, Atif S, Rauwerda J, et al. Endoscopic thoracic sympathectomy: long-term results for treatment of upper limb hyperhidrosis and facial blushing. Acta Chir Belg 2011;111:293–7.

27. Cameron AE. Specific complications and mortality of endoscopic thoracic sympathectomy. Clin Auton Res 2003;13(Suppl 1):131–5.

28. Drott C. Highlights from the discussions. Eur J Surg 1998;580(Suppl):47–50.

29. Li X, Tu Y, Lin M, et al. Endoscopic thoracic sympathectomy for palmar hyperhidrosis: a randomized control trial comparing T3 and T2-4 ablation. Ann Thorac Surg 2008;85:1747–51.

30. Yano M, Kiriyama M, Fukai I, et al. Endoscopic thoracic sympathectomy for palmar hyperhidrosis: efficacy of T2 and T3 ganglion resection. Surgery 2005;138:40–5.

31. Licht PB, Laadegaard L, Pilegaard HK. Thoracoscopic sympathectomy for isolated facial blushing. Ann Thorac Surg 2006;81:1863–6.

32. Walling HW, Swick BL. Treatment options for hyperhidrosis. Am J Clin Dermatol 2011;12:285–95.

33. Cruz MJ, Fonseca M, Pinto FJ, et al. Cardiopulmonary effects following endoscopic thoracic sympathectomy for primary hyperhidrosis. Eur J Cardiothorac Surg 2009;36:491–6.

34. Ouriel K, Moss AJ. Long QT syndrome: an indication for cervicothoracic sympathectomy. Cardiovasc Surg 1995;3:475–8.

35. Wettervik C, Claes G, Drott C, et al. Endoscopic transthoracic sympathicotomy for severe angina. Lancet 1995;345:97–8.

36. Drott C, Claes G, Göthberg G, et al. Cardiac effects of endoscopic electrocautery of the upper thoracic sympathetic chain. Eur J Surg 1994;572(Suppl): 65–70.

37. Drott C, Claes G, Rex L, et al. Long term effects of endoscopic thoracic sympathicotomy (ETS) for hyperhidrosis and facial blushing. Läkartidningen 2001;98:1766–72 [in Swedish].

38. Endoscopic thoracic sympathectomy for primary facial blushing. Available at: www.nice.org.uk/guidance/ipg480. Accessed August 23, 2015.

# Management of Plantar Hyperhidrosis with Endoscopic Lumbar Sympathectomy

Roman Rieger, MD

## KEYWORDS

• Plantar hyperhidrosis • Endoscopic lumbar sympathectomy • Retroperitoneoscopy

## KEY POINTS

• Primary plantar hyperhidrosis is defined as excessive secretion of the sweat glands of the feet and may lead to significant limitations in private and professional lifestyle and reduction of health-related quality of life.
• Conservative therapy measures usually fail to provide sufficient relieve of symptoms and do not allow long-lasting elimination of hyperhidrosis.
• Endoscopic lumbar sympathectomy is effective and safe in the treatment of plantar hyperhidrosis, which can be eliminated in more than 95% of cases with low morbidity and an acceptable rate of unwanted side effects.

## INTRODUCTION

Primary plantar hyperhidrosis is characterized by the excessive secretion of eccrine sweat glands of the feet. The etiology is unknown; however, a disturbance in the regulation of the sweat glands via the autonomous nervous system may play a role. In most times, the onset of the disease is in childhood or puberty but late onset in adults may occur. In more than half of the patients, plantar hyperhidrosis is associated with palmar hyperhidrosis.

The excessive sweating may be associated with cold and cyanotic skin, bromhidrosis, skin maceration, and bacterial and fungal skin infection and may lead to significant limitations in private and professional lifestyle as well as to physical and mental stress with potential reduction of health-related quality of life.[1–3]

Primary therapy includes hygienic measures, topical use of aluminum chloride and tannin-containing solutions, iontophoresis, and in selected cases botulinum toxin injections.[1,3] Although these measures may lead to a temporary relief of symptoms, they do not allow long-term elimination of the excessive sweat gland secretion.[4] Lumbar sympathectomy has been considered as a therapeutic option in severe cases of plantar hyperhidrosis because interruption of the sympathetic innervation of the eccrine sweat glands causes anhidrosis of the feet. However, the invasive nature of the procedure and the danger of significant unwanted side effects have prevented wide clinical application.[3]

In the following, we describe our experience with endoscopic lumbar sympathectomy for the treatment of patients with severe plantar hyperhidrosis.

## PATIENTS

From December 2004 until August 2015 a total of 188 patients underwent bilateral endoscopic lumbar sympathectomy for severe

Conflict of Interest: The author has nothing to disclose.
Department of Surgery, Salzkammergut-Klinikum Gmunden, Miller von Aichholzstrasse 49, Gmunden 4810, Austria
E-mail address: Roman.Rieger@gespag.at

thoracic.theclinics.com

plantar hyperhidrosis at the surgical department Salzkammergut-Klinikum Gmunden, Austria. There were 105 male patients and 83 female patients with an average age of 34 years (range 13–69). All patients had severe primary plantar hyperhidrosis that could not be controlled with conservative treatment methods such as the topical use of aluminum chloride solutions, iontophoresis, and in some cases botulinum toxin injections. A total of 75 of the patients (40%) had bilateral endoscopic thoracic sympathectomy for palmar hyperhidrosis 3 to 192 months previously.

## TECHNIQUE OF ENDOSCOPIC LUMBAR SYMPATHECTOMY

The surgical technique has already been described elsewhere in detail.[5] In brief, all procedures are carried out under general anesthesia and endotracheal intubation in supine position with hyperextended flank. To facilitate the localization of the various levels of the lumbar sympathetic trunk and its ganglia, the projection of the lumbar vertebral bodies onto the anterior abdominal wall is marked with fluoroscopy (**Fig. 1**). The procedure is carried out endoscopically with 3 trocars in the flank and continuous CO2 insufflation (see **Fig. 1**). The lumbar sympathetic trunk is presented at the level of the third and fourth lumbar vertebral body, whereby on the right side the caval vein and on the left side the para-aortal fatty and lymph node tissue must be dissected to medial. After the placement of metal clips to the cranial and caudal transection site, the segment of the sympathetic trunk situated between the clips is resected together with the ganglia L3 and/or L4 (**Fig. 2**). All specimens are sent for histology analysis.

## CLINICAL RESULTS

In several studies[6–8] we investigated the effectiveness and safety of endoscopic lumbar sympathectomy for the treatment of patients with primary plantar hyperhidrosis. The following section summarizes the results with respect to elimination of hyperhidrosis, morbidity and mortality, occurrence of unwanted side effects, rate of satisfaction of the patients with the postoperative result, and effect of the operation on quality of life.

It clearly could be shown that endoscopic lumbar sympathectomies can be performed with low morbidity and no lethality. Morbidity ranged from 3.0% to 4.6% and included only minor surgical complications like muscle or wound hematoma at a trocar insertion side as well as postoperative pneumonia in one and pulmonary embolism in another patient. Clinically relevant cardiovascular or blood pressure changes were not observed.[6,7]

So far, all operations were performed endoscopically, conversion to an open procedure was never necessary. There were no severe intraoperative complications; however, in approximately 25% of cases the endoscopic operation proved to be technically difficult due to a limited exposure of the retroperitoneum (most times due to the development of a pneumoperitoneum) or a difficult dissection of the sympathetic chain behind the vena cava.

In one study it was demonstrated that lumbar sympathectomy leads to an effective sympathetic dennervation of the blood vessels and the sweat glands of the feet. After the operation, the skin temperature of the sole increased an average of 2.8°C and transepidermal water loss of the feet was reduced significantly in all cases.[6]

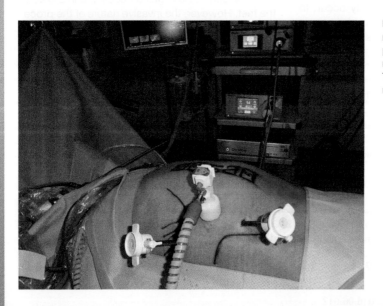

Fig. 1. Trocar placement during right-sided endoscopic lumbar sympathectomy. On 10 mm and two 5-mm trocars are placed in the flank. The lumbar vertebral bodies are marked on the abdominal wall.

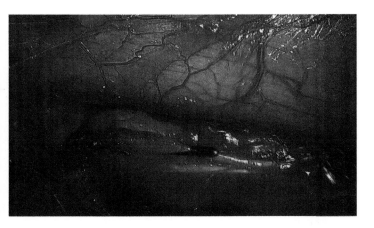

**Fig. 2.** Intraoperative view of the lumbar sympathetic chain behind the vena cava. Clips are placed on the sympathetic trunk superior and inferior to the third lumbar ganglion.

Immediately after the operation, hyperhidrosis was eliminated in all patients. In 2 studies with an average follow-up of 24 and 37 months, it could be shown that in most patients this effect was durable with anhidrosis of the feet in approximately 85% and slight remaining skin moisture in 12% of patients. Hyperhidrosis on one or both feet recurred in only 3% of patients between 1 week and 48 months after the operation.[6,7]

Unwanted side effects of the operation occurred in approximately two-thirds of the patients and included compensatory sweating (25%–44%) and postsympathectomy neuralgia (14%–42%). Compensatory sweating was minor in most cases and usually affected the abdomen and back, followed by hands, axillas, buttocks, and head. Postsympathectomy neuralgia usually occurred between the second and eighth postoperative day. The pain always disappeared spontaneously after 1 week to 3 months but lasted in a few patients up to 12 months.[6,7]

No patient so far suffered permanent sexual dysfunction, but in 3 men temporary loss or "weakness" of ejaculation occurred.

Most patients were very satisfied (73%–80%) or satisfied (17%–23%) with the postoperative result and 88% to 92% of patients would repeat the procedure.

In a recent study using the SF-36V2 questionnaire and 2 hyperhidrosis-specific questionnaires, we could demonstrate that severe primary plantar hyperhidrosis is associated with a reduced quality of life and that the performance of a lumbar sympathectomy leads to an increase of quality of life.[8] The SF-36V2 questionnaire revealed a significant improvement of quality of life after lumbar sympathectomy in the domains physical health (physical component summary) as well as mental health (mental component summary). Improved quality of life was also demonstrated in the Milanez de Campos questionnaire in the domains functionality/social interaction, intimacy, emotionality, and specific circumstances, as well as in the Keller questionnaire in the area of plantar hyperhidrosis.[8]

## DISCUSSION

The consequences of excessive sweating of the feet, such as unstable foothold in shoes, problems with walking barefoot, permanently cold feet, the appearance of painful skin lesions, and rotting of socks and shoes are often underestimated. Especially the bromhidrosis that occurs through the bacterial decomposition of sweat leads to a penetrating development of odor and thereby to enormous stress and stigmatization of the affected person. Although this clearly leads to a reduction of quality of life, the general public as well as many physicians consider plantar hyperhidrosis to be a trivial condition.

Primary treatment procedures such as consequent pedal hygiene, topical use of AlCl solutions, and iontophoresis can produce at least a temporary improvement of symptoms but usually proves to be ineffective in severe cases. The intradermal injection of botulinum toxin A has also been recommended for the treatment of plantar hyperhidrosis.[3,9,10] The efficacy of this treatment for plantar hyperhidrosis, however, has so far not been sufficiently proven by studies and has also not been greatly accepted by patients, because the injections into the sole of the foot are extremely painful, the effect of botulinum toxin is limited to a few months, and the necessary repeat applications are cost-intensive.

As plantar hyperhidrosis is associated with palmar hyperhidrosis in approximately 50% of cases, these patients frequently undergo thoracic sympathectomy. It has been reported that thoracic sympathectomy leads to a reduction of the sweat glands of the feet in as many as 42% of patients; however, most patients with severe plantar hyperhidrosis cannot experience sufficient improvement with thoracic sympathectomy.[11–13]

Interruption of the lumbar sympathetic trunk leads to sympathetic denervation of the sweat glands and blood vessels of the feet and in our experience, and also has been shown by other authors, plantar hyperhidrosis can be eliminated or clearly improved in 95% of patients by means of bilateral lumbar sympathectomy.[6–8,14–16] However, due to missing long-term observational studies, it remains unclear whether blocking of the sweat glands will persist in the long run.

Interruption of the lumbar sympathetic trunk can also be achieved with percutaneous application of alcohol, phenol, or radiofrequency, but experience with these techniques for treating plantar hyperhidrosis is limited. Although some optimistic results achieved with these methods have been reported, considerable doubts remain as to long-term efficacy.[17,18] Compared with conservative procedures, permanent elimination of the condition can be achieved with lumbar sympathectomy, which is why, similar to thoracic sympathectomy, the procedure has the potential for high acceptance in patients despite the existing risks.

Acceptance of the procedure as well as quality of life and satisfaction with the postoperative result correlates closely with the risks of the surgical procedure and the intensity and frequency of unwanted side effects.[19,20] Although it could be demonstrated that endoscopic lumbar sympathectomy can be performed with low morbidity, the potential risks of this operation must not be underestimated. Especially the dissection of the lumbar sympathetic trunk behind the caval vein and in proximity to lumbar vessels can be a challenge and harbors the danger of problematic bleeding. This risk must be viewed critically in relation to the indication for the procedure.

Like after thoracic sympathectomy, unwanted side effects, such as compensatory sweating and postsympathectomy neuralgia, occur frequently after lumbar sympathectomy and were the main reasons for dissatisfaction with the result of the operation. However, in contrast to thoracic sympathectomy, severe compensatory sweating is rare after lumbar sympathectomy and occurred in only 2% of our patients.[6,7]

Potential sexual dysfunction disorder in men has led to a widespread rejection of lumbar sympathectomy for the treatment of plantar hyperhidrosis.[3] In the few available historical studies that included almost only patients who underwent lumbar sympathectomy for peripheral arterial occlusive disease, ejaculation disorders have been reported between 0.8% and 54% and were usually observed only if the upper lumbar ganglia have been included in the sympathectomy of at least one side but especially of both sides.[21–23]

Our experience indicates that permanent ejaculatory dysfunction can most likely be avoided when lumbar sympathectomy is limited to the level of the third or fourth lumbar vertebral body. However, due to the considerable anatomic variability of the autonomous nervous system in the lumbosacral region, sexual dysfunction after lumbar sympathectomy probably can never be ruled out completely.

## SUMMARY

Endoscopic lumbar sympathectomy appears to be a safe and effective procedure for eliminating excessive sweating of the feet and improves quality of life of patients with severe plantar hyperhidrosis.

## REFERENCES

1. Eisenach JH, Atkinson JLD, Fealey RD. Hyperhidrosis: evolving therapies for a well-established phenomenon. Mayo Clin Proc 2005;80:657–66.
2. Tetteh HA, Groth SS, Kast T, et al. Primary palmoplantar hyperhidrosis and thoracoscopic sympathectomy: a new objective assessment method. Ann Thorac Surg 2009;87:267–74.
3. Hornberger J, Grimes K, Naumann M, et al. Recognition, diagnosis, and treatment of primary focal hyperhidrosis. J Am Acad Dermatol 2004;51: 274–86.
4. Moran KT, Brady MP. Surgical management of primary hyperhidrosis. Br J Surg 1991;78:279–83.
5. Rieger R, Pedevilla S. Retroperitoneoscopic lumbar sympathectomy for the treatment of plantar hyperhidrosis: technique and preliminary findings. Surg Endosc 2007;21:129–35.
6. Rieger R, Pedevilla S, Pöchlauer S. Endoscopic lumbar sympathectomy for plantar hyperhidrosis. Br J Surg 2009;96:1422–8.
7. Rieger R, Loureiro MP, Pedevilla S, et al. Endoscopic lumbar sympathectomy following thoracic sympathectomy in patients with palmoplantar hyperhidrosis. World J Surg 2011;35:49–53.
8. Rieger R, Pedevilla S, Lausecker J. Quality of life after endoscopic lumbar sympathectomy for primary plantar hyperhidrosis. World J Surg 2015; 39:905–11.
9. Haider A, Solish N. Focal hyperhidrosis: diagnosis and management. CMAJ 2005;172:69–75.
10. Vadoud-Seyedi J. Treatment of plantar hyperhidrosis with botulinum toxin type A. Int J Dermatol 2004;43: 969–71.

11. Rieger R, Pedevilla S, Pöchlauer S. Therapie der palmaren und axillären Hyperhidrose-Thorakoskopische Resektion des Truncus sympathicus. Chirurg 2008; 79:1151–61.

12. Andrews BT, Rennie JA. Predicting changes in the distribution of sweating following thoracic sympathectomy. Br J Surg 1997;84:1702–4.

13. Neumayer CH, Panhofer P, Zacherl J, et al. Effect of endoscopic thoracic sympathetic block on plantar hyperhidrosis. Arch Surg 2005;140:676–80.

14. Reisfeld R. Endoscopic lumbar sympathectomy for focal plantar hyperhidrosis using the clamping method. Surg Laparosc Endosc Percutan Tech 2010;20:231–6.

15. Loureiro Mde P, de Campos JR, Kauffman P, et al. Endoscopic lumbar sympathectomy for women: effect on compensatory sweat. Clinics 2008;63: 189–96.

16. Nicolas C, Grosdidier G, Granel F, et al. Endoscopic sympathectomy for palmar and plantar hyperhidrosis: results in 107 patients. Ann Dermatol Venereol 2000;127:1057–63.

17. Nickel J, Jahnel A, Andresen R. CT-gestützte lumbale Sympathikolyse bei Hyperhidrosis plantaris. Rofo 2004;176:122.

18. Kim WO, Yoon KB, Kil HK, et al. Chemical lumbar sympathetic block in the treatment of plantar hyperhidrosis: a study of 69 patients. Dermatol Surg 2008; 34:1340–5.

19. Jaffer U, Weedon K, Cameron EP. Factors affecting outcome following endoscopic thoracic sympathectomy. Br J Surg 2007;94:1108–12.

20. Panofer P, Zacherl J, Jakesz R, et al. Improved quality of life after sympathetic block for upper limb hyperhidrosis. Br J Surg 2006;93:582–6.

21. Rose SS. An investigation into sterility after lumbar ganglionectomy. Br Med J 1953;1:247–50.

22. Whitelaw GP, Smithwick RH. Some secondary effects of sympathectomy. With particular reference to disturbance of sexual function. N Engl J Med 1951;245:121–30.

23. Quayle JB. Sexual function after bilateral lumbar sympathectomy and aorto-iliac by-pass surgery. J Cardiovasc Surg 1980;21:215–8.

# Index

*Note:* Page numbers of article titles are in **boldface** type.

thoracic.theclinics.com

# UNITED STATES POSTAL SERVICE®

## Statement of Ownership, Management, and Circulation
(All Periodicals Publications Except Requester Publications)

| | | |
|---|---|---|
| 1. Publication Title | 2. Publication Number | 3. Filing Date |
| THORACIC SURGERY CLINICS | 013 – 126 | 9/18/2016 |

| | | |
|---|---|---|
| 4. Issue Frequency | 5. Number of Issues Published Annually | 6. Annual Subscription Price |
| FEB, MAY, AUG, NOV | 4 | $350.00 |

7. Complete Mailing Address of Known Office of Publication (Not printer) (Street, city, county, state, and ZIP+4®)

ELSEVIER INC.
360 PARK AVENUE SOUTH
NEW YORK, NY 10010-1710

Contact Person
STEPHEN R. BUSHING

Telephone (Include area code)
215-239-3688

8. Complete Mailing Address of Headquarters or General Business Office of Publisher (Not printer)

ELSEVIER INC.
360 PARK AVENUE SOUTH
NEW YORK, NY 10010-1710

9. Full Names and Complete Mailing Addresses of Publisher, Editor, and Managing Editor (Do not leave blank)

Publisher (Name and complete mailing address)

LINDA BELFUS, ELSEVIER INC.
1600 JOHN F KENNEDY BLVD. SUITE 1800
PHILADELPHIA, PA 19103-2899

Editor (Name and complete mailing address)

JOHN VASSALLO, ELSEVIER INC.
1600 JOHN F KENNEDY BLVD. SUITE 1800
PHILADELPHIA, PA 19103-2899

Managing Editor (Name and complete mailing address)

ADRIANNE BRIGIDO, ELSEVIER INC.
1600 JOHN F KENNEDY BLVD. SUITE 1800
PHILADELPHIA, PA 19103-2899

10. Owner (Do not leave blank. If the publication is owned by a corporation, give the name and address of the corporation immediately followed by the names and addresses of all stockholders owning or holding 1 percent or more of the total amount of stock. If not owned by a corporation, give the names and addresses of the individual owners. If owned by a partnership or other unincorporated firm, give its name and address as well as those of each individual owner. If the publication is published by a nonprofit organization, give its name and address.)

| Full Name | Complete Mailing Address |
|---|---|
| WHOLLY OWNED SUBSIDIARY OF REED/ELSEVIER, US HOLDINGS | 1600 JOHN F KENNEDY BLVD. SUITE 1800 PHILADELPHIA, PA 19103-2899 |

11. Known Bondholders, Mortgagees, and Other Security Holders Owning or Holding 1 Percent or More of Total Amount of Bonds, Mortgages, or Other Securities. If none, check box. ► ☐ None

| Full Name | Complete Mailing Address |
|---|---|
| N/A | |

12. Tax Status (For completion by nonprofit organizations authorized to mail at nonprofit rates) (Check one)
The purpose, function, and nonprofit status of this organization and the exempt status for federal income tax purposes:
☐ Has Not Changed During Preceding 12 Months
☐ Has Changed During Preceding 12 Months (Publisher must submit explanation of change with this statement)

| | |
|---|---|
| 13. Publication Title | 14. Issue Date for Circulation Data Below |
| THORACIC SURGERY CLINICS | AUGUST 2016 |

| 15. Extent and Nature of Circulation | | | Average No. Copies Each Issue During Preceding 12 Months | No. Copies of Single Issue Published Nearest to Filing Date |
|---|---|---|---|---|
| a. Total Number of Copies (Net press run) | | | 382 | 488 |
| b. Paid Circulation (By Mail and Outside the Mail) | (1) | Mailed Outside-County Paid Subscriptions Stated on PS Form 3541 (Include paid distribution above nominal rate, advertiser's proof copies, and exchange copies) | 143 | 174 |
| | (2) | Mailed In-County Paid Subscriptions Stated on PS Form 3541 (Include paid distribution above nominal rate, advertiser's proof copies, and exchange copies) | 0 | 0 |
| | (3) | Paid Distribution Outside the Mails Including Sales Through Dealers and Carriers, Street Vendors, Counter Sales, and Other Paid Distribution Outside USPS® | 100 | 128 |
| | (4) | Paid Distribution by Other Classes of Mail Through the USPS (e.g. First-Class Mail®) | 0 | 0 |
| c. Total Paid Distribution (Sum of 15b (1), (2), (3), and (4)) | | ► | 243 | 302 |
| d. Free or Nominal Rate Distribution (By Mail and Outside the Mail) | (1) | Free or Nominal Rate Outside-County Copies included on PS Form 3541 | 42 | 61 |
| | (2) | Free or Nominal Rate In-County Copies Included on PS Form 3541 | 0 | 0 |
| | (3) | Free or Nominal Rate Copies Mailed at Other Classes Through the USPS (e.g. First-Class Mail) | 0 | 0 |
| | (4) | Free or Nominal Rate Distribution Outside the Mail (Carriers or other means) | 0 | 0 |
| e. Total Free or Nominal Rate Distribution (Sum of 15d (1), (2), (3) and (4)) | | ► | 42 | 61 |
| f. Total Distribution (Sum of 15c and 15e) | | ► | 285 | 363 |
| g. Copies not Distributed (See Instructions to Publishers #4 (page #3)) | | ► | 97 | 125 |
| h. Total (Sum of 15f and g) | | ► | 382 | 488 |
| i. Percent Paid (15c divided by 15f times 100) | | ► | 85% | 83% |

* If you are claiming electronic copies, go to line 16 on page 3. If you are not claiming electronic copies, skip to line 17 on page 3.

| 16. Electronic Copy Circulation | Average No. Copies Each Issue During Preceding 12 Months | No. Copies of Single Issue Published Nearest to Filing Date |
|---|---|---|
| a. Paid Electronic Copies ► | 0 | 0 |
| b. Total Paid Print Copies (Line 15c) + Paid Electronic Copies (Line 16a) ► | 243 | 302 |
| c. Total Print Distribution (Line 15f) + Paid Electronic Copies (Line 16a) ► | 285 | 363 |
| d. Percent Paid (Both Print & Electronic Copies) (16b divided by 16c × 100) ► | 85% | 83% |

☒ I certify that 50% of all my distributed copies (electronic and print) are paid above a nominal price.

17. Publication of Statement of Ownership
☒ If the publication is a general publication, publication of this statement is required. Will be printed in the NOVEMBER 2016 issue of this publication. ☐ Publication not required.

18. Signature and Title of Editor, Publisher, Business Manager, or Owner

STEPHEN R. BUSHING - INVENTORY DISTRIBUTION CONTROL MANAGER

Date 9/18/2016

I certify that all information furnished on this form is true and complete. I understand that anyone who furnishes false or misleading information on this form or who omits material or information requested on the form may be subject to criminal sanctions (including fines and imprisonment) and/or civil sanctions (including civil penalties).

PS Form **3526**, July 2014 (Page 3 of 4)   PRIVACY NOTICE: See our privacy policy on www.usps.com.

PS Form **3526**, July 2014 (Page 1 of 4 (see instructions page 4))   PSN: 7530-01-000-9931   PRIVACY NOTICE: See our privacy policy on www.usps.com

Printed and bound by CPI Group (UK) Ltd, Croydon, CR0 4YY

08/05/2025

01864692-0005